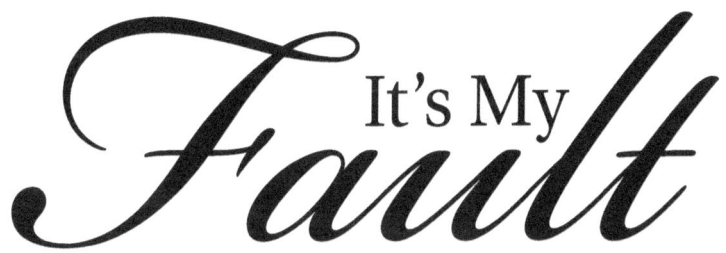

It's My Fault

My Journey through Breast Cancer

SHERRY KAY THOMPSON

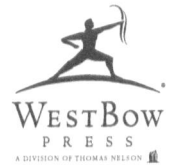

WESTBOW
PRESS
A DIVISION OF THOMAS NELSON

WestBow Press books may be ordered through booksellers or by contacting:

WestBow Press
A Division of Thomas Nelson
1663 Liberty Drive
Bloomington, IN 47403
www.westbowpress.com
1-(866) 928-1240

Author photo by Jen Arney Photography.

Cover photo by Jessica Brankamp.

ISBN: 978-1-4908-0700-3 (sc)
ISBN: 978-1-4908-0699-0 (hc)
ISBN: 978-1-4908-0701-0 (e)

Library of Congress Control Number: 2013915817

Printed in the United States of America.

WestBow Press rev. date: 09/13/2013

Dedication: Thank you to the young man that jumped in the swimming hole in his church clothes on Shurz Road in Middletown OH and saved me from drowning when I was around five years old. I don't know your name but I thank you with all of my heart.

Don't expect everyone to understand your journey, especially if they've never had to walk your path!
Anonymous

Table of Contents

The Beginning

S A TEENAGER I always thought I wanted to be like the women they talked about in magazines who used their breasts as a source of "power over the opposite sex." Who were these ladies? The girls I knew in high school who used their breasts to get male attention were what some people referred to as sluts. Some girls used theirs just to tease guys however I do not recall the girls I knew using them to have power over the opposite sex. This is not a politically correct thing to think or say anyway having power with your breasts!!! However back then the idea of having power over men was something I thought I wanted. I felt like the boys in school had too much power over us so I wanted something that would give me power to level the playing field. Even if it meant I had to use my breasts to get there! I guess it is for the best I never found out how to use my breasts as sources of power over men because having power with your breasts is no real power at all.

I have had a long and bumpy ride with my breasts. I developed breasts earlier than most of the girls I knew and I spent lots of time hiding my breasts or trying to figure out why they caused such odd reactions from both genders. As the HealthDay News says, "For many girls, an overly large cup size may not be such a good thing, with many reporting serious discomfort both physically and emotionally because of their large breasts." The first "emotionally discomforting" incident I recall happened right after I first developed breasts. I was in fourth grade and a girl whom I had never spoken to yelled this as I walked by, "No mine are bigger than hers." This girl thought she had won a competition that I did not even know I was competing in. When I moved to a new school in fifth grade I had developed size "B" cup breasts. I was quite popular with the boys. The popular girls wanted to befriend me since I was getting the boys attention. This did not last long once they realized how shy I was and how my strict mother would not let me go to any of the parties to which they tried to invite me. I remember one girl begging me to be her friend and once I was no longer "popular" the same girl acting like I had the plague. What power did these breasts have and why did I hate the attention they brought me?

In sixth grade I was walking on the playground with my best friend and some boys yelled out, "She stuffs her bra those things are falsies." I was shocked and hurt. "What did that mean?" I wondered, and why did they say that to me. Why had they said this to me and not my friend Kathy who was walking with me? I had to be told by my wise and worldly friend (can a sixth grader really be worldly?), what the boys had really meant. I asked her if there was anything I could do to prove these breasts were part of my body and not socks stuffed in my bra. She said, "They are yelling at you because they want you to show them your breasts." Well I was not going to be showing them anything. One of the boys who yelled the insult at me had man-boobs bigger than mine because he was overweight. Why could one of the fattest and ugliest boys at school feel like it was okay to yell crude things to me? Why didn't I tell him he was fat, ugly and mean? Because I was shy and was not mean like he was I kept my mouth shut and stayed away from those rude boys. Did my breasts and I have to take rude remarks and do nothing? I started wearing a tent-like dress (I looked like I had a maternity dress on) to hide my breasts. I think I wore it twice a week. The dress put me in a comfort zone my other normal fitting dresses and tops did not. Unfortunately I could not wear it every day. I became very cautious and fearful. I began to doubt myself wondering, "Maybe I was causing these insults by flaunting my breasts."

When I was younger I had not learned to think of my breasts as assets. Even though they brought me lots of attention, I did not like the type of attention I got. One day in eight-grade, I was walking down the hall laughing with a friend and a popular middle school female classmate yelled, "How embarrassing for her she cannot even stuff them evenly." She was the most popular girl in school why did she care about me? My friend said the girl was just jealous. I asked myself, "Why didn't I yell something back at her?" I told myself I could not stand up to her because she was surrounded by her group of in-crowd friends and all I had with me was one friend. My friend was just as afraid as I was of the popular kids. This particular popular girl was notorious for bullying anyone who was not in her clique or up to her "standards." So instead of having a witty come back for the loud mouthed popular girl I gave her a death stare and ran to the bathroom to look in the mirror. I checked to see if what the "junior high critic" had said was true, were my breasts oddly uneven? Had they become misshapen since I left home this morning, no they looked the same as the last time I had looked at them. Why did my breasts always insist on causing me so many problems? Why did I let a loud mouthed bully make me doubt myself? Why did the adults I knew act like it was my fault if someone was crude or rude to me regarding my breasts? Why did they try to insinuate if I had been born a boy or had been born a female with smaller breasts then I would not have problems with men? I know lots of women are taunted and abused who have small breasts and I know boys who have been abused and taunted. People have said things to me which made me feel inferior and guilty about the way my body looked because I was born a female with large breasts.

One of my uncles tried to make me feel inferior because I was a child of adoption. When I was about 14 years old, I was supposed to go visit my older sister and spend the night. My brother had said he would take me to her house. He seemed annoyed and put out because he had to drive me there. An uncle was at our house visiting, he rarely visited so it was odd he was even there. He offered to take me to my sister's house since it was only a few minutes from where he lived. I was hesitant because I did not know him well. I was hoping my brother would say, "Oh no I promised Sherry I would take her." But he seemed relieved he did not have to take me to my sister's house. I was surprised my mother agreed to let my uncle take me to my sister's house because she kept a tight leash on me and always said, "You cannot trust men or boys." She agreed so off we went to my sister's house. On the way he asked me about being adopted. He said, "Your parents really do not love you like they do their own kids because you are adopted." I could not figure out why he was saying those mean things. Later I thought about what he had said and wondered, "Was he right? Did my parents not love me as much as they would have if I had been a child of their loins and not an adopted child?" I think my uncle was a mean person and just wanted to make me feel bad about myself. When you are a teenager something an adult says to make you feel inferior really shakes you up. In my case adults made me feel bad about my breast size and my uncle made me feel bad that I was adopted. Being a teenager is confusing enough as it is, adults should be careful because teens take things like that to heart and believe what an adult says.

When I was a teenager my younger sister begrudgingly used to say, "You look like a Barbie doll but your breasts are saggy." However the reason they were "a little saggy" was because they were so full and large. Rude guys were always trying to feel my breasts to "see if they were real." One guy friend told me what he thought was a compliment he said, "When describing you I said you were the one with the big breasts and they immediately knew who you were." I did not think what he had said to describe me was a compliment and I was shocked he and other people thought of me as "the one with the big breasts." I was much more than the size of my chest! I was Sherry, on some days I felt pretty, some days I felt shy, and some days I liked my breasts even though they obviously were not what other people thought of as the "proper" size. I also was Sherry who loved to laugh and who got good grades and loved Home Economics. My teacher was sweet and once said a lavender skirt and white blouse I had on looked like it came straight out of a fashion magazine because I had placed a lavender scarf around my neck to "make the outfit." My teacher had not mentioned my breasts and she loved my outfit. I had a tendency to let moments like that one be tainted by crude comments made by thoughtless, hurtful people. I remember one such incident in my high school art class when a former elementary boyfriend said to another guy, "Oh my god I do not think she has a bra on." We were walking out of class and they were behind me. He knew I could hear what he said but I was too shocked to turn around and reply. I wanted to say, "Well I do have a bra on and thanks for making me never want to wear this shirt again. Also my crush on you is now finished." I wanted to be remembered for more than my breast size. The question was would I ever be more than that to some people? If those people focused on only one part of my body then they were not the type of people I should care about. When someone said something crude to me, made a snide remark to my face or "whispered" something rude within my earshot, I never had a good comeback. Would a snappy comeback have been my saving grace?

I had been brought up in a strict and ultra-religious family with parents who believed parts of the body like breasts should not be discussed. I never felt like I could ask anyone in my family the question, "Why are my breasts getting guys attention?" My family felt if a person got attention with a body part it was somehow their fault. I knew from past experience if I told my mother what was happening to me she would tell me I was to blame. She would say, "Well look how you dress. You're too skinny and guys like skinny girls." Or she would say, "What did you say or do to make young men say those things to you?" I know anything I said about the problems I had because of my breast size would be turned around to be my fault. Once I started dating I knew the guys I wanted to date found my breasts quite interesting (I followed their eyes), however I wanted to be thought of as anything else than "the girl with big breasts."

Even after I graduated from High School and got married there were many times when I felt my breasts were the only thing about me a lot of people found interesting. I hated it when I walked down the street in a mid-calf raincoat and still got cat-calls. It just did not make sense to me. I was not wearing a low-cut top or tight clothes, I had on a raincoat for goodness sake. So why was it okay for men to yell nasty comments at me? Why couldn't I just shrug off these comments and love myself and my breasts? Why was I not more like a relative of mine who lived for cat calls from men? Well actually I could never be like her because I did not find cat calls from random strangers or even from the local yokels flattering or endearing. Not only did my breasts cause unwanted attention from strangers they also caused me to have lots of back problems. The first time my back went out was when I was 17 and working at McDonalds. The doctor I saw after my injury informed me my back would always cause problems because I was so tall and had such large breasts. So now not only were my breasts objects of ridicule and obscene comments they now were causing my back to "go out."

Even though I did occasionally have back problems sometimes I loved my breasts. If I found a certain blouse or shirt that fit well I thought they looked amazing. When I did find a top which fit well I wanted to wear it every day. I once found a swimsuit which looked perfect. It was a bikini and it actually covered my breasts. They had started selling bikini bottoms separate from bikini tops. I could buy a medium top and a small bottom and they both fit. Previously when I purchased a two-piece swimsuit I had to buy the same size top and bottom as a set. I usually had to worry about the suit either being too big on the bottom if I bought a medium suit or my breasts popping out if I bought a small swimsuit. This swimsuit was perfect and when my hubby and I went to a park for a family picnic and played volleyball in the pool I felt comfortable in my own skin. I was 20 and do not remember ever feeling this comfortable with my body in a swimsuit. It was a wonderful feeling.

I became a mother and breastfed both of my daughters and I thought of my breasts differently. I now thought of my breasts more as tools. They were tools that provided food for my babies. I wondered if other people thought of them the same way. Would they be thought of less as sexual objects and therefore less of a problem? When a friend made a snide remark telling me her hubby liked her smaller boobs because he said big boobs make women "look like cows." I realized my breasts were still causing problems. I realized she was jealous and trying to make me feel bad about the way I looked! I secretly envied her smaller size chest because she could wear anything she wanted to wear. I always felt I had to wear loose tops or ill-fitting tops. Were my breasts always going to be a source of problems?

The older I got the more I accepted my breasts because they did not seem to bring as much attention as they did when I was younger. I continued to have back problems due to my heavy breasts and I continued to see a chiropractor. I also saw a back specialist and my MD on a regular basis. The sessions with my chiropractor helped ease my back pain but as I got older I gained a lot of weight which caused my breasts to get bigger and my back to hurt more. I decided to get breast reduction surgery when I was in my early 50's. I had gained a lot of weight and instead of having nice double "D" size breasts I had matronly size double "E" breasts. I tried to diet and I also tried to exercise the fat away but my large breasts just always seemed to get in the way. I was happy with the size of my breasts after my breast reduction surgery. The doctor told me he took 5 pounds of fat from each breast. The scars were minimal and the recovery time was not terrible either so once again I was pleased with my breasts.

A Travel Business

M Y DAUGHTER SHAWNDRA and I opened a sports travel business and took our first group on a trip in July 2010. These trips require a lot of pre-planning with my overseas contacts and I also have to get a lot of information from the teams for my airline contact. Once we get to the international location the group has chosen we are busy keeping 20 or more people happy. We have to stick to a pretty strict schedule and follow our planned itinerary. Free days are built into each schedule and are a lot more relaxing. We always have to be available to the group even if we have a free day scheduled. Our first trip was to Athens, Greece. We were lucky because our daughters got to travel with us. My youngest even brought her husband. My daughters run the travel business with me so I wanted them to come with us on our first trip. We stayed in Athens the majority of the trip in a little boutique hotel right downtown. We saw the Parliament and the changing of the guards on the first night we were there. In the proceeding days we toured the Parthenon and the Temple of Zeus and went to the Plaka neighborhood for dinner. The Greeks refer to Plaka as the neighborhood of the Gods. We ate outdoors on the rooftop and had an amazing meal. We also ate dinner the next night at an outdoor restaurant that had a view of the Acropolis fully lit up which gave it a surreal look. We had toured the Acropolis during the day but at night it was quite magical all lit up. For the second part of our trip we took a four hour bus ride to Kalamata (the town is named after the olives). The Greek hillsides and small towns were breathtakingly beautiful. Once we got to the four star resort we were pleasantly surprised. It had a huge pool and the staff was at our beck and call because the hotel was pretty empty. It was quiet and had an amazing view of the Aegean Sea. Our room was in the back of the complex and when we walked to our room we could smell jasmine which grew on an arch-shaped trellis over our heads. It smelled like what I imagine heaven will smell like. Kalamata was a wonderful change of pace from Athens.

The people in the small town of Kalamata were much happier and laid back so we felt a lot more welcomed there than we had in Athens. The women's basketball team we were chaperoning played one game in this small town and the whole town seemed to be there to watch the game. We got to swim in the Aegean Sea while we were there and see one of the most beautiful sunsets I have ever seen in my life. When I travel to an international location I am reminded of this quote: "I cannot think of anything which excites a greater sense of childlike wonder than to be in a country where you are ignorant of almost everything," Bill Bryson. I think that quote really describes perfectly why I love to travel abroad it does give me a childlike sense of wonder and we all need that childlike wonder in our lives.

The Bad News

*A*FTER OUR WONDERFUL business trip to Greece we did a family road trip to Washington D.C. It was in September 2010 and we went to a rally for Union workers (my husband is a union worker and we were there to support the union and to give the union a voice). Some governors were trying to dismantle unions, (including the Governor of the state we lived in). My husband's union wanted to have a large number of union members attend this rally to let the people who governed us know we did not approve of their tactics to destroy unions. I had never been to Washington D.C. before and was so excited to go with my hubby and my youngest daughter Jessie. After the rally we also went to Chinatown, saw the Lincoln memorial, took pictures in front of the White House and did a ton of other touristy things. We were having so much fun exploring Washington D.C. My youngest had been there one time before with her eighth grade class so she loved being our tour guide and telling us all the things she remembered about her previous trip.

During all this fun and family time, I got a call from my gynecologist. I listened to my voice message and it was not a nurse it was my doctor saying, "Please call I need to talk to you about your mammogram results ASAP." I had been seeing him for more than 20 years and more than once I had to go back to get a repeat mammogram because the first one "was not clear." So when I had to get a follow up mammogram this time I had not thought twice about it. This time was different obviously because my doctor had never called before. When my doctor left three messages on my phone during my weekend trip, I knew it was not good news. I did not want to call back and as I told my husband, "It cannot be good news because the doctor never calls, only his nurses call." My husband insisted I was over reacting. He called the doctor's office while I went into a store and distanced myself from him. I did not want to over-hear the phone call. After my husband called the doctor he found me in a souvenir store and I could tell from his face the news was not good. The doctor told my husband that the mammogram had shown two spots on my breast. He said he needed me to schedule a biopsy and see a general surgeon as soon as I returned home.

I had a biopsy preformed and it was not as easy as I had been told it would be. I had to lay face down while the surgeon was under me performing the biopsy. It was awkward because I was not put to sleep. My breasts were hanging down out of a table with an opening cut in the table especially for the breasts. My head was to the side. They gave me epinephrine and I had a bad reaction to it so we had to stop in the middle of the surgery. I was shaking and crying and could not stop. The nurse told me I was having a bad reaction and they would give me a different drug when they resumed the surgery. After I settled down they resumed the surgery with a different drug and things went smoothly after that. A few days later my husband went with me to see the general surgeon my GYN had recommended and he told us he had the biopsy results. He said he had "good news" I did not have cancer however I had to have my breast removed. When is getting a breast removed ever considered good news? He said I was lucky because the aggressive pre-cancer (or as they call it Stage zero cancer) was caught in time and did not go to my bones or move to other parts of my body. He said I was lucky. I did not feel lucky. I was glad he thought my chances looked good. I did not like the doctor telling me how the news about having my breast chopped off was good news! As my friend Brenda George said in her book <u>Rejoicing Through The Tears</u>, "There is no good cancer. Cancer can kill. It may be slow, depending on what type it is and the stage it is in, left untreated, death is almost inevitable. The "C" word is one nobody ever wants to hear. The very word meant death to me. If I was fortunate enough to survive, my life would be forever changed . . ."

Even though my surgeon said he was delivering good news it was not good news. I was losing a breast. I knew it was great they thought they had caught the cancer before it moved to another part of my body or into my bones. I did not appreciate it when my surgeon acted like I should be smiling from ear to ear about his "good news." My husband and I were in shock we both felt like we had taken a hard blow to the stomach. My husband kept asking questions as I sat in quiet shock with no words to form into sentences. When I did finally form words I asked the doctor, "Will I be able to spare my nipple?" I had read in a magazine at my GYN's office that sometimes when removing a breast the patient could still keep her nipple intact. The doctor said, "No the nipple was leaking and had pre-cancer cells in it so it could not be spared." He also told us we needed to "calm down." Funny I had not noticed we were not calm. So apparently we were having a bad reaction to his "good news" and he did not approve? The way the doctor treated me did not seem like a normal way for a doctor to treat a patient who was going to lose one of her breasts. Where was his sympathy or at least empathy? We left his office in shock and we both walked around in a daze for the next few weeks. My husband and I had already planned a week in Florida before this "good news" so we went down to our Florida vacation home and while we were there I did some research on the type of cancer the doctor said I had. He said the type of pre-cancer I had was called DCIS.

Surgery

*I*FOUND A definition of DCIS on the internet from the Mayo Clinic Staff it said: Ductal carcinoma in situ (DCIS) is the presence of abnormal cells inside a milk duct in the breast. DCIS is considered the earliest form of breast cancer. DCIS is noninvasive, meaning it hasn't spread out of the milk duct to invade other parts of the breast. DCIS is usually found during a mammogram done as part of breast cancer screening. Because of increased screening with mammograms, the rate at which DCIS is diagnosed has increased dramatically in recent years. While DCIS isn't life-threatening, it does require treatment to prevent the condition from becoming invasive. Most women with DCIS are effectively treated with breast-conserving surgery and radiation. I wondered, "If this was true why was the doctor recommending that I have a mastectomy?" I also found out there was an option I should consider. Maybe I should get both breasts removed instead of one. Statistics show women who have cancer in one breast have a 50% higher chance of getting cancer in their other breast than women who have never had breast cancer. So when I returned from Florida I asked my surgeon two questions: "Why was a getting a mastectomy surgery if what I had read on the internet was true about DCIS normally being controlled by "breast conserving" surgery followed by radiation?" And, "Could I get both breasts removed?" His answer to the first question was, "Because you have multiple pre-cancer spots inside the milk duct breast removal is the safest way to go." Regarding having the second breast removed he said, "The insurance company will not pay to have the second mastectomy." So I proceeded to get only my left breast removed. I was terrified to have my breast removed I tried to be strong for my family. My oldest daughter flew up from Savannah to be at my side. My youngest daughter's hubby David even took the day off and they drove up from their home in KY to be at my side. My allergies were bad that day so the nurse gave me a breathing treatment before my surgery. I kept up a good face and tried to joke and laugh a lot while my family encircled my bedside. But my oldest daughter told me that once they gave me a sedative and rolled me down the hall I cried non-stop. All my grief came pouring out once the sedative pulled down my defenses. I do not remember crying or anything else that happened once they put the sedative in my IV until I woke up in pain after the surgery. The doctor tested the lymph node tissue that he had removed during surgery to make sure cancer had not spread. He told my family that the cancer had not spread to my lymph nodes and I did not have to have chemo or radiation therapy treatments. My family took me home. I was in severe pain. When I tried to move from one couch to the other I passed out from the pain. I remember feeling a searing pain and the feeling that my chest was being ripped open. When I woke up Mark was standing over me patting my face and saying my name over and over. It was a terrifying experience. I decided I did not want to go through that again so I crawled up the steps and pulled myself onto the bed. My husband and my son-in-law tried to help me but I screamed "NO!" I told them I was afraid if they lifted me up the searing pain in my chest would come back and I would pass out cold again. My youngest took care of me and my husband did too until he had to go back to work.

Once I was on my own I lay in the bed and cried with my cats around me. My stomach was upset and my back was killing me because the medicine from the IV they had inserted during surgery made me severely constipated. Whenever I get constipated my back goes out so I was in a lot of pain. I walked around on the third day after my surgery crying and singing because it was too painful to sit down. When I finally had a bowel movement by the fourth day it hurt so much I thought I might die on the commode. I also had drainage tubes in my body and they smelled funny, which meant no matter how many showers I took or how much perfume I wore, I smelled funny. I had to stuff my bra because I was flat on the left side of my chest. It hurt to wear stuffing because my surgery wound was still very tender and painful. I wore only sports bras because regular bras seemed too tight and when I added stuffing it was very uncomfortable, and painful. I really felt awful and was not much fun to be around. I worried about the future surgeries I had to have and I worried if my husband would accept the "new me." I did have some good things happen during this time. My friend Jennifer whom I use to work with stopped by and brought me quiche, salad and dessert, all the fixings for a wonderful meal. Also Harold and Jean, a couple we knew, brought by dinner and homemade bourbon ice cream for dessert. They are quite the bourbon enthusiasts and the ice cream was amazing! When everyone went back to their normal lives and I had to be alone I realized I could not go back to my normal life. Would my life ever be normal again? I was sad and lonely. I tried to think positive thoughts however sometimes I was just so depressed.

On my worst days my cats and I would stay in bed all day and right before my husband came home from work I would get up and shower so he would not know I had been in bed all day, sad and depressed. Thank goodness I had my cats to keep me company. They were a constant source of comfort to me when I was sick or blue. I think the only way I got out of my funk was by thinking about our future trip to Florida for my birthday and our Anniversary which we had planned. I always looked forward to traveling. But now I was really looking forward to getting out of the cold weather and going to the sunshine state. I was leaving my sadness behind in Ohio and going to happy, sunny Florida. We had a wonderful Florida trip and when I got home I visited my daughter Jessie every week or she came to see me and I continued working on a trip we were taking to Italy for our sports travel business. I was busy collecting information from the coach about the team we were taking to Italy and relaying the information to my international vender there. It was good to have something to keep me busy and another trip to look forward to going on. Time flew by and my daughter Jessie and I were busy planning to go on the trip to Italy. My husband was traveling with us and my daughter's husband was thinking about joining us too. She found out in the summer she was pregnant and could not go on the business trip. She was disappointed because she could not go but very excited that she was newly pregnant. I was also excited to be a grandmother.

Before my husband and I took the Women's basketball team on our trip to Italy my doctor had scheduled saline implant surgery. My general surgeon could not do saline implants. He had noticed the breast reduction scar on my remaining breast and had commented on what a great job the plastic surgeon had done. So the general surgeon recommended that I should get the same plastic surgeon to preform my saline implant surgery. The surgery was performed by my plastic surgeon and was much easier on my body. The saline injections which followed were extremely painful because my skin was being stretched to make room for a silicone implant. I would be getting a silicone implant put in sometime in the month of December for now I was stuffing my bra with washcloths. I needed to find a bra which would camouflage the saline implant. It was sitting very high on my chest and did not match my regular breast. I went shopping at a store especially for women with breast cancer. They fitted me with a bra and stuffed it with silicone breast forms to try and match my saline breast with my real breast. I was shocked when the total price was $1700.00. They assured me the insurance would pay for most of the cost. My insurance company ended up only covering $700 of the bill.

I did not know the insurance would not cover the cost. If I would have known I would not have made the purchase. I proceeded to shop for my trip using advice I received from the clerk at the breast cancer store. She said to, "Buy blouses with big designs on them to "camouflage any imperfections the bra and breast forms cannot hide." I went shopping for our trip to Italy and before I knew it August first had arrived. It was time to travel to Italy.

Our first stop was a little hotel right outside of Venice. We then took a ferry to Venice and visited St. Mark's Basilica and toured St. Mark's square. On the way back to our hotel our ferry stopped at Murano Island for a glass blowing demonstration. I purchased some hand blown wine stoppers for gifts. During our first evening in Italy, we held a clinic in Rovigo which ended with a scrimmage against male and female players. Our women's basketball team and about 40 locals took a pic for the clinic that was well attended by Rovigo locals. After the game we went to a local restaurant and some of the Italian coaches and other adults that had attended the clinic as observers where there. They bought champagne for the team and we had so much fun talking with them while we shared a meal. To our surprise the clinic that the team had put on for the local kids was featured in three local newspapers the next day!

Our next stop was a little known place called San Marino. The bus had to wind through steep hills and curvy roads to get there. San Marino is the third smallest country in Europe, with only Vatican City and Monaco being smaller. San Marino has no natural level ground; it is entirely composed of hilly terrain. The views were amazing and our hotel rooms were in what looked like a castle. After one night there we headed to a small town outside of Florence called Montecatini Terme. We stayed in this wonderful small town for three nights. It was close enough to Florence that we could hop on the train and be in there in 30 minutes. The second day we hopped on the train and headed to Florence. We then got on the hop on hop off bus to and rode up to the Piazzale Michelangelo. It overlooks Florence from its perch in the hills high above the city. A fake statue of David and a little café are located there. We sat and drank wine and soaked up the view. While we were in Florence we also made sure to sample the Gelato because the locals say Florence has the best Gelato in all of Italy. The last three days of the trip were spent in downtown Rome. My favorite sight in Rome was the church inside Vatican City called St. Peters Basilica. I felt so humbled by the Holy history of the beautiful cathedral. We came back to Vatican City at night via a double decker bus and got to enjoy the view of the city all lit up. It was quite a sight to behold. While I was on the double decker bus with the breeze in my hair I thought, "Life does not get any better than this." The people, the sights and the food were wonderful and I would like to return one day on a trip with the family. We were gone a total of eleven days. During the trip we were busy the entire time making sure the games were on time, and the team got to the excursions that my vender had arranged for them. Last but not least we wanted to make sure the team, coaches and parents had fun. I was exhausted when we got home however the memories and the beauty of Italy kept me going.

After we returned from Italy I began to do research on normal procedures that breast cancer patients follow. I found out most cancer patients see an oncologist before they see a general surgeon. I wish I would have been able to see an oncologist prior to my surgery. I would have liked surgery options explained to me before making a final decision with a surgeon. An oncologist might have given me the option of having a lumpectomy which would have involved having my two pre-cancer spots removed from my breast, followed by radiation or chemotherapy. An oncologist might have also given me the option of removing my second breast at the same time I had the first breast removed. Instead I was sent to a general surgeon who did not give me any of those options. When we are patients we do not know what steps are next. We believe what our doctor tells us and we are at their mercy. I wish I would have seen an oncologist before my first mastectomy. I did not and there is nothing I can do about it now. The results may have been the same, I still may have had to get a mastectomy however I would have liked to been told my options.

I also started doing research on various movie stars who had dealt with breast cancer. I was waiting for an appointment at my plastic surgeon's office when I found a free cancer magazine with Christina Applegate on the cover. In her teen years she had starred in the TV show "Married with Children," which I had watched religiously back in the day. In the article she discussed her cancer journey. I took the magazine home and looked up info about her on the internet. Applegate was still an actress currently starring in the TV sitcom, "Up all Night" in spite of the fact that she had gotten both of her breasts removed due to cancer. It was inspiring to read Christina's cancer story. A TV news entertainment anchor, Giuliana Ranic, recently announced she had been diagnosed with breast cancer and was going to undergo a lumpectomy followed by chemo and radiation therapy because the doctor's had found two spots in her breast. I found this very relatable because I had also been diagnosed with two spots in my breast. The doctor's performed the surgery but later decided she needed to undergo a double mastectomy. They said the lumpectomy had not gotten all the cancer spots. She also had implants put in immediately following her double mastectomy surgery. I always wondered why I was not given the option to have my two spots removed instead of a mastectomy so the news about Giuliana having a cancer diagnose similar to mine, made me think that maybe my mastectomy was the right decision after all. Her experience with breast cancer was so similar to mine and she had gone through it and came out whole and happy. It gave me hope and I was so glad she had shared her experience and did not hide it from the public. Sheryl Crow is another celebrity who has been very vocal about her breast cancer. She now has a non-malignant tumor in her brain. But she said after going through her breast cancer experience this tumor is just a bump in the road. During her cancer journey she was so brave and strong. I also read in Louis-Post Dispatch about ABC morning show host Robin Roberts who battled breast cancer and survived.

Unfortunately she now has to deal with MDS, a condition which affects bones and bone marrow. She developed an aggressive form of the disease as a result of her breast cancer therapy several years ago. Roberts left the morning show to have chemotherapy and a bone marrow transplant to fight her myelodysplastic syndrome. Her doctor said "I want to emphasize this is a rare complication and a rare event. Most women with breast cancer have a much higher risk of breast cancer returning than developing MDS." It is always scary to learn how the very treatment which cures a person's breast cancer can be the cause of another serious illness. The doctor said what happened to Robin was rare. She is a strong lady and I know she will get through this second round of illness. I admire all these women because they have been so brave during their illnesses. They have shown such a love of life and such a desire to get to the other side of their illnesses. They have shared their experiences with breast cancer and it gives women like me lots of hope and encouragement.

Besides doing internet research on celebrity breast cancer survivors, I was also busy updating my business website with travel blogs and pictures of our trip to Italy. I made photo discs of the trip for my family. I knew I had one more surgery to go through in December. I was not dreading it like I had been before the trip. The trip to Italy had made me more willing to live life and not lay in bed depressed and feeling sorry for myself. I put the thought of surgery right out of my mind and began looking forward to birth of our first grandbaby.

In September I planned a baby shower for my daughter, Jessie. I was crazy busy painting the family room and painting some old furniture I was putting into the room. My husband moved out the furniture which had previously been in the room and moved in different couches and end tables. I planned the menu for the baby shower for weeks and cooked the food with help from my oldest daughter Shawndra who drove up to our house to attend the baby shower. The shower was a roaring success. They say the true sign of a successful party is if the hostess has fun. If she is having fun, then most likely the guests are also. Well the guests must have had a blast because I did. Balloons and baby banners decorated the freshly painted recreation room and all the guests took home a goody bag. In the goody bags we had a mini bottle of liquor, a recipe for the cupcakes I made for the shower (it was the cake I craved when I was pregnant with Jessie), candy and other goodies. Everyone raved about the quiche and chocolate peanut butter cheesecake I made for the shower and we also had lemon scones, chocolate cupcakes, salad and iced tea. My oldest was the photographer for the party snapping away pictures and capturing the special moments with the new fancy professional camera we had just bought her for her freelance writing business. Jessie got great gifts. She also had fun posing with her husband for pregnancy pictures. My oldest daughter Shawndra took the pregnancy pictures with her new camera after the shower. I was on a happy high from the shower for months. I was so grateful to all the people who attended the shower and I felt like a new woman.

I was also looking forward to a cruise to Australia my husband had planned. I think my husband was trying to go to all the places we have always wanted to go but never had the time or money to go to before. Since my cancer diagnosis we have embraced Mark Twain's philosophy about life. Twain said, "Twenty years from now you will be more disappointed by the things you did not do than the ones you did. So sail away from the safe harbor. Catch the trade winds. Explore, Dream. Discover." We also wanted to scope out the location because many colleges had shown an interest in traveling to Australia. So as Twain suggested we went on our next adventure a cruise to Australia.

We had planned this cruise to celebrate my one year "cancer free" anniversary. When we got back from our cruise I would have a new grandbaby to hold in my arms. Our trip in November to Australia was as they say "an adventure of a lifetime." I had to be very careful with what I wore because my saline implant was high up on my chest and did not match the "real breast." The expensive forms I bought from the breast cancer store made my back hurt because they were too heavy. I instead used some inexpensive foam forms I had found via a catalog at my plastic surgeon's office. The way my saline implant sat so high on my chest made it hard to wear a swimsuit. I always had to wear foam inserts in my bra to make my breasts match. I decided I would wear my sheer cover-up anytime we went to a beach because the cover-up seemed to hide any imperfections my swimsuit did not hide. I tried to forget about my breast issues and have a great time. The year had been a rough one with a saline implant surgery followed by four painful saline injections designed to stretch out my breast skin to ready it for a silicone implant. Followed by months of waiting for the skin to stretch out and accept the new shape. I was excited because I would be getting a silicone implant soon however I was dreading the surgery. When we flew to San Francisco to begin our adventure I was really looking forward to the trip and to getting my mind off of my breast issues.

Eighteen Days on a Cruise Ship

*T*HE CRUISE LINE had included in our cruise package, airfare from San Francisco to Honolulu so we flew to San Francisco two days early so we could explore the city before we took the cruise leaving from Honolulu. While we were in San Francisco we explored Fishermen's Wharf and the Golden Gate Bridge. We also rode the hop on hop off bus and got to see a lot of wonderful sites. We saw the crooked street named Lombard everyone talks about. We also went through the Haight Ashbury area where the Flower Children lived back in the 60's and 70's. I love Jimi Hendrix and there is a mural of him and a lot of other singers from that particular era. They sang about free love and experimented with mind expanding drugs. The hop on hop off bus also drove by the house featured in the TV series "Full House." It was in a beautiful neighborhood across from a huge park. I really loved everything about San Francisco. On our last morning there we went to the Ghirardelli Chocolate factory and watched them make chocolates. We drank Ghirardelli hot chocolate and bought some souvenirs. It was so relaxing and fun. It was a nice way to spend the last day in San Francisco.

We had been to Honolulu in 2006 when our oldest daughter Shawndra worked for another travel company. She was chaperoning a team of college age women volleyball players. We got to see a lot during that visit including Waikiki Beach, Diamond Head, North Shore and the Brigham Young College where the girls played against the BYC women's college volleyball team. I liked this trip much better because we did not have to worry about staying with the team or attending the volleyball games like we did in 2006. On this trip we were glad we got to see Pearl Harbor because we had missed it on our previous trip to Honolulu. It made my heart ache to know that a ship full of sailors went down on that very spot. It was unnerving to learn that the ship and sailors were still buried under the very memorial building we were standing on.

We loved our two days in Honolulu and we were looking forward to getting on the cruise ship and seeing more of Hawaii. We found out on our last day there the President was coming to town and the traffic was going to be backed up if we did not leave early. There were secret service agents at our hotel and they had shut down an elevator for some important dignitaries who were staying there. I kept hoping I would see the President. We did not get to see the President however we did have a wonderful time. I called the cruise lines to see if we could get on our ship early to avoid traffic and they told us we could come aboard any time after 11am. We got on board about noon. I was so excited to get on the cruise ship which would take us on our 18-day cruise. The view of Honolulu from the top deck of the ship was amazing. Our first port of call was Maui. We did an excursion to the highpoint of the island and saw breathtaking views all along the way. After we left Maui we traveled for five days at sea to the port of Papeete. It was a beautiful island. I was shocked to see how poor a lot of the people appeared to be. I think traveling is good for Americans because we get to see that other people live a very different kind of life. It makes me very happy that I live in America.

During the next three days we traveled to the Tahitian islands of Mariena, Raiatea and Bora Bora. These islands were amazing. The waters were the most beautiful colors I had ever seen and the people were friendly. We took one excursion to a small unnamed island and we went snorkeling and saw colorful fish and amazing coral. It felt like we were in paradise. The next day we did an excursion to another unnamed island. We stayed three hours eating locally made food and freshly caught fish. We also swam and explored the island. I sat under a shade tree drinking beer with my feet dangling in the cool water while Mark swam over to a nearby island and did some exploring. I really felt at peace and can now understand why people love the South Pacific so much.

We set sail for our next leg of the trip, eight days at sea. We started appreciating how nice our ship was. Our cabin was so cozy and we had gotten upgraded for free to the Concierge deck with a balcony. Because we were on the Concierge deck we received two free bottles of champagne on our arrival and fresh flowers and appetizers brought to our room every night. We really felt pampered. I loved the Celebrity X ship because it was a smaller ship than any I had ever been on and the food and service was amazing. I also ordered an internet package so I could email our daughters and keep in contact with some friends. We signed up to attend two events while we were at sea. The first event we attended was wine tasting in the afternoon. It was so much fun and we learned how the size and type of wine glass a person uses makes a lot of difference on how the wine tastes. The other event we attended was High Tea. I wore a dress and Mark wore a suit to the Tea. They served champagne and had a harp player and a pianist. The food was so good. Even though I did not think my husband would like the tea he said he did. Both events cost extra however it was so much fun to try something new. We kept busy doing crossword puzzles and reading. We also went to the gym and worked out. Mark did various exercises for an hour a day and I worked out on the elliptical machine for a half an hour each day. There were also a lot of free activities planned on the ship such as sushi making, touring the kitchens and bingo. Even though we did not try any of the activities is was great to have those options. We usually went down early and had a drink before dinner in the lounge and we always got the same waitress. We loved her and I had Mark take my picture with her so I could post it on Facebook. When we took the picture all her co-workers laughed and said, "You are going to be on Facebook." She was also the person we ordered drinks from when we were in the dining room and she was usually our cocktail waitress when we went to see a show.

While we were on the cruise we ate dinner with the same people every night because we were assigned to a dinner table. We met a nice couple whose names were Harriet and Richard. Richard even borrowed a suit jacket from Mark for the formal dinner nights. He had not brought a suit jacket and on formal night men were required to wear them. He did not want to miss a single night of dinner with our group. Mark lent him one of the three suit jackets he had bought especially for our cruise. They make cat toys for a living and when we returned home they promised they would send us toys for our cats. There was also a fun mom and son at our table from Australia (the husband had to cancel at the last minute due to an illness so the son filled in). A third couple rarely came to dinner preferring to eat in their room or eat at the self-serve buffet.

We looked forward to dinner every night and after dinner we would go the shows provided on the ship. There were usually dancers, comedians and sometimes even a Broadway style show. One night they had Polynesian style dancers and they were picking people out of the audience to dance with them. When a male dancer came up and asked me to dance I froze then I said, "Yes." You have to realize I am one shy lady and would have rather done almost anything than get up on stage and dance. When I went up there and danced I was so nervous I do not remember anything except that it was fun.

Our next port was Sydney so we asked the mother and son who sat at our dinner table and were from Australia what to do and see while we were there. They suggested we ride the hop on hop off bus and they said we needed to try the famous meat pies. After being at sea eight days we arrived at the Sydney Harbor at about 4am. Because the ship was small we could hear the noise from the anchor being hauled in and the sound of the tugboat horns and every other noise involved in bringing a ship to port. Due to all the noise I woke up at 4:30am. I took pictures of the Harbor and the famous Opera House. The city was still asleep and it looked beautiful surrounded in a light fog. It was so exciting to be in Australia. We stayed in Sydney two days and fell in love with the city. The cute little boutique hotel where we stayed was very close to the hop on hop off bus stop. The bus took passengers on a tour of downtown Sydney and it also took us out of town to Bondi Beach. We ate meat pies (a local specialty) and went to Bondi Beach and toured the entire city. The locals were so friendly and it was nice to speak the same language. I loved the accent they had when they spoke. The two days in Sydney flew by and then we took a flight with Qantas airlines back to San Francisco. I was dreading the flight because I have always heard how awful it was to fly from Australia to the USA because it is such a long flight.

We were pleasantly surprised because we were up in the exit row with no one in front of us so we had tons of leg room and could get up without bothering anyone. The wine was free and we had our own screens to watch a choice of about 20 movies. We both got up to stretch a lot and took a few naps and before we knew it we were back in San Francisco. Once we got there we spent the night at a hotel then flew home the next day. We were gone for a total of three weeks. I really did not get homesick the whole time. I missed my daughters and my cats and I was ready to go home even though we really had a great cruise. When we got home I watched the video of myself dancing with the Polynesian dancer. I laughed my head off. When we showed it to the kids they thought it was funny too. Oh my! My dancing was an experience to remember and something I can laugh about now. At the time I thought I was going to pass out from stage fright. The male dancers were dressed in very skimpy costumes and they were quite young and handsome. If nothing else I can always brag a buff young man asked me to dance while we were on our trip.

I had my silicone implant surgery in December when we got back from our cruise and the day after my surgery our grandson was born. I thought waiting for the birth of our grandson at the hospital would be too hard on me because I had just had surgery. However because my surgeon had only had to make a small incision to remove the saline implant and put a silicone implant in its place, the recovery time and the pain afterwards was nothing like my first mastectomy. He had also put anti-nausea medicine in my IV to prevent me from getting sick to my stomach or getting constipated. It was amazing because it worked. I was in no pain during the 12 hour wait for my grandson to be born. I was thrilled when he was born and I got to hold him. What a precious bundle of joy he was. I realized soon after my surgery that the silicone implant did not match the "real" breast I still had. But at least now I could wear a wider range of clothes. If I wore blouses with designs or flowers on them people would not notice I had one breast one size smaller than the other or that one breast sat higher on my chest than the other. I did not mope about my breasts not matching for too long because I had a sweet baby grandson to hold in my arms, a website to update, listing Australia as our special trip that year and a trip to Las Vegas in February to celebrate my birthday and our anniversary to look forward to. I was feeling good and things were looking great.

The good feeling went away when I started having pains in my right breast. I was now on my second oncologist. I had quit going to the first oncologist because I felt she rushed me through appointments and made a sick face when she first saw my breast cancer scar. I liked the fact that she was female however I did not like her bedside manner so I asked my plastic surgeon to recommend another oncologist. This oncologist was male and he was wonderful on the first visit. He took a lot of time discussing my issues and I thought he is going to work out great. When I began to have pains in my right breast I was worried. I wondered, "Did I have cancer in my right breast?" I went to the oncologist to ask him about the odd pains I was having in my right breast. He said,

"The pains you are having is just normal pains because you had a breast reduction two years ago." He saw me for less than two minutes and his nurse said, "Oh he is behind schedule so we need to keep him on track today." I was not happy with his diagnosis. He did not order any tests. He just assumed a diagnosis without even thinking twice which was not good enough for me. I had gone to him because I was not happy with my first oncologist now he was displaying the same behavior my first oncologist had by rushing me through my appointment. I knew my chances to get breast cancer in my right breast were higher than the average woman because once a woman has had breast cancer in one breast they are 50% more likely to get it in the other breast than a woman who has never had breast cancer. After the terrible rushed appointment with him. I made the decision to try and see my original oncologist. When I went to see her about the breast pain I was having she scheduled an MRI. I was relieved because at least she wanted to run tests. I began to wish I would have never changed oncologists. After having an MRI I received the results which showed I had lesions and irregular cells. So the oncologist set up a Biopsy to confirm the MRI test results. I got the biopsy done and hoped for the best.

In the meantime we flew to Las Vegas in February of 2012 to celebrate my 56th birthday and to also celebrate our 38th anniversary. We were staying in a condo and we would be there ten days. We rented a car and bought groceries when we got there, then we planned what we wanted to see while on our trip. We had always stayed downtown on our previous trips to Las Vegas and we had never rented a car. On this trip we were on the North side of the strip away from the casinos. It would have been a long walk to the strip or a long ride on the bus if we had not rented a car. We also needed a car because we wanted to travel outside the city limits to Zion National Park and Lake Mead. We spent the first couple of days sleeping in and going to the casinos. Neither of us does much gambling however we do love to see the sites like the water show at the Bellagio Casino and the Volcano show at the Mirage. We also went to the Mirage to see the Beatles Cirque De Soleil show. One night we saw a comedian by the name of Vinnie Favorito, at Harrah's casino. When we bought the tickets for Vinnie's show the lady at the counter warned us his humor was raunchy and he picked on audience members however he was hilarious! We were lucky he did not pick on us. We were sweating when he got to the row in front of us. Thankfully his show ended before he got to us. The humor was so politically incorrect but we still laughed our heads off.

We also went to the Cosmopolitan Casino so I could have one of their specialty drinks called the White Cosmo. Toward the end of our stay we headed to Zion Park in Utah and The Valley of Fire just outside of Las Vegas. The views were breathtaking on the drive to the park. They were also amazing once we got inside the park. It was so weird we had never been outside of Vegas we had always stayed downtown and missed the beautiful world outside of the city lights. After being in a crowded city full of lights the mountain drive was eerie at night with the darkness and emptiness. I loved the mountains during the day but at night there were just too many miles of nothing but pitch black darkness and very few houses or any kind of civilization.

We loved the condo in Las Vegas because we could make our own meals and be lazy and watch TV till the afternoon if we wanted to. I found some yummy cinnamon bread and made French toast with it for breakfast on quite a few mornings. We also found some choice steak at the local market and I made steak and onions quite a few times. We did go out to eat a lot too however it was fun to have the option of making our own meals. We experienced Las Vegas in a way we never had before.

We tried not to think about my biopsy results during our Vegas trip. We just wanted to have fun and not worry about anything. One thing which did make me worry during the trip was the repeated phone calls I kept getting from my MD. I missed the calls every time because we were so busy in Vegas and I did not hear my phone ring or I had it turned off. After the third message from my MD's office I called to find out what was going on. I called the office and the nurse said the biopsy had come back inconclusive. She said I needed further testing. She said to contact my oncologist. I called my oncologist and was told by her nurse they had not gotten the test results yet. I told her it was odd she had not received the results because they were sent to my MD already. The nurse said she would look into it and call me the next day. She called the next day and said, "The doctor said the tests came back fine and she will see you next year." I was so happy about the news, even though in the back of my mind I thought it was odd my MD's office had said just the opposite. When we got home I got a letter in the mail from the place that did my last tests. The letter stated I needed more tests done on my right breast and I should call my oncologist. I called my oncologist and they again informed me nothing was wrong with me and I did not need any further tests. At this point I was very confused because my MD and the office where my biopsy had been performed were telling me my tests showed irregular cells and lesions in my breasts and I needed further testing. Why was my oncologist telling me something completely different?

The Doctor Said What?

WHEN I GOT conflicting info from my oncologist I decided to make an appointment with my GYN. He was the one who originally told me about the cancer in my left breast maybe he could sort out all the conflicting information I had received. I went to see him two months after my original test results were sent to me. He was his normal kind and caring self. He answered all the questions my husband and I threw at him and he decided I needed to see the same general surgeon who had performed my first mastectomy. Needless to say I was not thrilled to see the same surgeon again because I was afraid I would be told I was too emotional like he told me the first time I saw him. But I decided because my GYN was such a good doctor, I would heed his advice. When I saw the surgeon he made sure to tell me the first oncologist (he had recommended her) had not read the tests wrong. He said her staff had "given her the wrong info." I decided to take the high road and said, "I do not feel comfortable seeing her again so it does not matter," I wondered in the back of my mind if he was doing this because he was afraid I was going to sue the oncologist he had recommended or if he was afraid I might sue him too. Because he started the appointment by defending the oncologist it made the appointment very awkward but somehow we muddled through.

He proceeded to tell me I had two options: I needed to get more tests ran and another biopsy done or I needed to get a mastectomy done on my right breast and insurance would pay for it. "Why was my insurance going to pay for the surgery," I asked. He said they would pay for my second surgery because I was considered a high risk for breast cancer since my left breast had breast cancer. This did not make any sense he was the doctor who said two years ago "Insurance will not pay to remove your second breast," yet he was now telling me they would pay for it.

I asked him if putting a silicone implant in during the surgery would be possible. I told him I had done research and talked to some friends about getting an implant put in the same time I had the mastectomy done. During my research and conversations with friends I discovered many women now choose this option if they do not need chemo or radiation. The insertion of a silicone implant immediately after the mastectomy saves women from additional surgeries and the pain of saline injections. He acted offended and said, "I do not do that type of surgery and if you get a plastic surgeon to perform the surgery the insurance will not pay for it." Well that was interesting he was saying the same thing he had said two years ago "insurance will not pay for it."

After seeing this surgeon who I did not like or trust, a horrible sad feeling came over me and I cried all the way home. I feel lost and alone. I went home and again did a lot of research. If I chose to get tests done instead of surgery, I would have to have tests done every six months. The tests would include a biopsy and/or MRI's depending on what the doctors thought I needed. I could not stand the thought of more tests especially tests every six months for who knew how long? I had been through a lot since my 2010 mastectomy. I had dealt with a rollercoaster of physical and emotional issues after I had my first mastectomy. I feared the future because it felt like every time I turned around I had a new surgery scheduled. The pain of the first surgery left me sick and weak and after a long recovery all I had to look forward to back then was more surgeries if I wanted to get a silicone breast implant. Once I decided I did want the silicone breast implant I first had to get a saline implant, followed by saline injections and then the silicone implant was put in. I tried to put on a good front however sometimes I just felt like all the pain was not worth the results. I could hardly bear the thought of one surgery let alone multiple surgeries. What was I going to do? Would I find a doctor who cared about me?

The next week I thought over my options and decided to make an appointment with my plastic surgeon. I thought my plastic surgeon could answer my questions and recommend a general surgeon who would put in a silicone implant immediately after the mastectomy, a surgeon who would perform one surgery instead of multiple surgeries. When I saw my plastic surgeon he said he could do the mastectomy with an immediate implant. He was not only a plastic surgeon he was a general surgeon so he could do both!! He said because there were many spots (lesions) in my breast that waiting six months to do further testing would only put off what needed to be done now. He asked me about my first cancer on the left breast. I told him they found two spots. He said this was why my breast was removed instead of just the spots being cut out when I had my first mastectomy. He said a lot of times when more than one spot appears on the biopsy results the doctor decides it makes much more sense to remove the breast than cut out the spots. He went on to say sometimes when only the spots are cut out all of the cancer is not removed. Then the surgery has to be repeated. He also said sometimes when they cut into a spot it divides and instead of one spot the surgeon then has two to spots to remove. It was reassuring to know I did the right thing by having my first mastectomy. I have had many negative comments from various friends and family regarding my first surgery. Comments such as, "Why not just get the spots removed, you did not really need mastectomy surgery," and, "A lumpectomy would have been so much less painful and invasive." What he told me seemed to dispel all the theories from people who had told me my decision to have my first mastectomy was the wrong thing to do. He said he would make sure this mastectomy surgery with an immediate silicone implant put in was approved by my insurance company. A week later his office called to schedule the surgery because the insurance company had approved my surgery. I was happy that my insurance had quickly approved the surgery but I wondered, "Why would my general surgeon refuse to work with a plastic surgeon? Why would he want me to have two surgeries instead on one?" I knew when my general surgeon did the first mastectomy he did not want to reschedule my surgery when I asked him to. Also when I asked him about the possibility of getting my second breast removed he said, "We already have the surgery to have just one breast removed scheduled and we will just stick with that schedule." He also said, "Insurance will not pay for that." I believe he thought his time was more important than me or my illness. I also had the answer to another question that kept swirling around in my head, "Why did he tell me a plastic surgeon could not do the surgery because the insurance company would not pay for it?" My plastic surgeon answered that question. He said general surgeons cannot legally do silicone implants however sometimes they work with a plastic surgeon and the mastectomy is done by the general surgeon then the plastic surgeon steps in to put in the silicone implant. Did the general surgeon just not want to work with a plastic surgeon? I guess I will never know the answer to that question because I decided that I was not going to use the general surgeon. I was never going to see him again. Instead I chose to use my plastic surgeon and I felt I was in good hands with him.

I was naïve when I got my first mastectomy but now I was much wiser and chose my plastic surgeon to do my second mastectomy. My plastic surgeon was a general surgeon and a plastic surgeon. He had done my breast reductions, my saline implant, my saline injections and my silicone implant on my left breast and I trusted him. I think this is very important when a person has cancer. A person needs a doctor that they like and a doctor they can trust. I was going to have to have another mastectomy but this time I was going to have the surgery performed by a doctor I trusted and liked. In the meantime we decided we would still go to Spain to celebrate the fact I was still alive because some good doctors had been diligent and followed up on my test results. We were also going there to check out the location for a future trip for our travel business. So we went on a cruise to Spain.

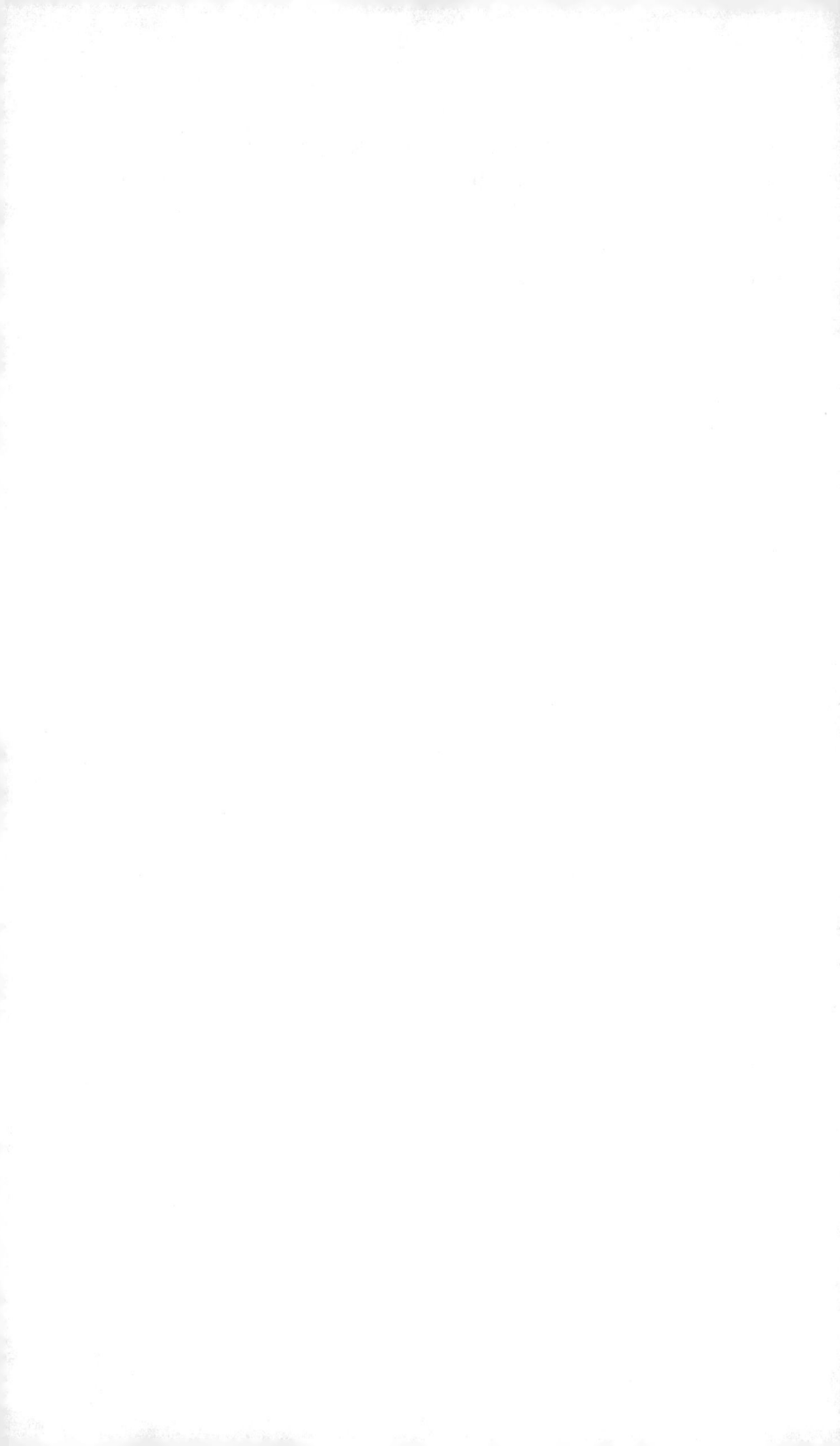

Spain

I WAS GLAD we had booked a cruise to get away from reality and get my mind off of my upcoming surgery. In April we flew to Miami, Florida and got on a cruise ship to Spain. I did not put on a swimsuit because the weather was chilly but some people still sat around in their swimsuits trying to tan if the sun even peaked out for a minute. Mark and I did not even hot tub because it was so chilly and the hot tubs were always so crowded. One day it was warm enough for Mark to try the amazing slides they had on board. I took pictures of him while he played on the slides. I was not comfortable enough with my uneven boobs to even put on a swimsuit to go down the waterslides.

We cruised past Bermuda and talked about how much fun it would be if the boat ported there. We did port at an island in Portugal and we went on an excursion which took us all around the island. We saw a Pineapple farm and went to some local shops. We also saw two lakes which were former volcanoes and at the top of these former volcanoes there were skydivers jumping off the top of the hills and floating down to the valley below, it was amazing to watch. On the way to Spain our ship went past the Rock of Gibraltar. Everyone went to the top deck so they could see the view. On the other side of the ship was a huge mountain in

Africa. It was gray colored and just so stunning to look at. I actually liked the view of the mountain more than the Rock of Gibraltar. People we taking all kinds of pictures and we took some pictures for couples who wanted to pose with the Rock of Gibraltar behind them and people took a few pictures for us.

We did not exchange phone numbers or addresses with anyone on this cruise because dining tables were not assigned so we did not sit with anyone. We had a table all to ourselves every night. We meet a nice couple when we first got on the ship while we were eating lunch. We went to a Margarita tasting event and meet a nice couple there. We sat and talked to them and drank for a while. We also sat by a nice couple at one of the shows and we talked during the show. I missed the wonderful dinners with the same group of people and the dinner conversations we had on the last cruise. One of my favorite parts of the last cruise was sitting with the same people every night at dinner.

The shows on this ship were wonderful. They had Blue Man Group, Cirque De Soleil Dinner and Dreams, Second City Comedy Club, a Blues Club and a group called Legends (it is a group of celebrity impersonators). At the Blue Man Group show one of the Blue Men came up to Mark and gave him some candy. He then indicated he wanted Mark to throw it at him. The Blue man tried to catch it in his mouth. Mark kept trying to make the Blue man miss the candy. The Blue man caught it every time! The skit was funny because of the facial expressions the Blue man made. They are a group who performs mime comedy so they do not speak. It is all physical comedy. At the end he gave Mark the candy he had chewed up it was a big wadded up ball of white chocolate and he wanted Mark to let him spit it in his hand. Mark would not let him spit it in his hand. Instead he gave the Blue man a cup to spit it in. It was hilarious. We saved it and when we got home we gave it to our son-in-law David who loves the Blue Man Group. He loved it. It still had some blue paint on it from the Blue man's hand. I told our son-in-law to sell it on E-bay. He decided to keep it as a souvenir.

Even though the entertainment was great on the big ship I think I liked the smaller ship on our previous cruise because of the assigned dinner seats, the fun of having the same people to eat with and the personalized service. Although one thing I really liked about this bigger ship was the Irish Pub. Passengers could go there for breakfast, lunch or dinner at no extra charge. At the pub they had a huge screen with movies showing a couple times a day so it was a fun place to eat and catch a movie. I bought an internet package so I could keep in contact with family and look at pictures of my grandson which my daughter Jessie frequently posted. The cruise was ten days long with just one port stop. When we got to Barcelona we were eager to get off the ship and onto land. We stayed in Barcelona two days. While we were there we did the hop on hop off bus and saw the town. It was a beautiful town with beaches on one side and hillsides on the other. The hotel we stayed at was the downtown Hilton and the people at the hotel all spoke English. We were exhausted the first day so we ate a late lunch at our hotel. We had a great waiter, the food was yummy and I tried some delicious Spanish wine. Our hotel was amazing and everyone was so friendly we even got upgraded to a suite and got free breakfast every morning and a manager special in the afternoon was also included. The manager special served appetizers and free beverages including wine and beer so we scheduled our day around the manager special so we could eat "dinner" free. It was so much easier to go to the hotel to eat than it was to hunt for a place to eat in town. Not only was the food free the dining area was located on the top floor of the hotel and it had a wonderful view of the city.

While we were sightseeing we saw tons of buildings designed by the famous architect Gaudi. He really created some unusual designs. One place where the bus dropped us off looked like a Dr. Seuss house. Gaudi was definitely an original and they are very proud of him in Barcelona. The second day we did the tour bus again and drove by Gaudi's Sagrada Fimilia cathedral with its three facades. The line was too long at the cathedral to go inside but we were amazed to see a church that has been under construction since 1892! We also bought some souvenirs and found a Subway shop where we ate lunch. After two days in Spain we flew back to the US. We landed in Fort Lauderdale and spent one night there then flew home. I missed home and my new grandson so much. The trip was exciting however it was good to be home.

We had taken the cruise to Spain so I could get my mind off my breast issues and check the location out for my tour company. However now that I was back home all I could think about was getting my second mastectomy surgery. Even though this mastectomy would be done in one surgery and it wouldn't be followed by multiple surgeries for a saline implant and a silicone implant like my previous mastectomy, I was still dreading having the surgery done. I had been through so much pain mentally and physically I really could not wrap my head around another surgery. During the following weeks before my surgery I tried to keep as busy as possible. I sorted through pictures of our Spain trip and I updated the business website listing Spain as our special trip that year. I also went to visit our grandson and daughter Jessie at least once a week. My grandson was growing and he was such a joy to be around. When I was with him he made me forget all my troubles.

One Nurse's Opinion

NE PERSON WHO did not help me forget my troubles was a registration nurse at the hospital where I went to get "pre-registered" for my second mastectomy a week prior to the surgery. The registration nurse asked, "Would you like to have the local breast cancer support group contact you after your surgery?" I said yes so she proceeded to fill out a paper with long laborious pen strokes and asked lots of personal questions. Her last question (which I know was not a question on the form) was, "Why is a plastic surgeon doing your surgery, will he have a general surgeon assisting?" I answered, "No he will not." She went on to say, "I have never known this Dr. to do mastectomies because he does not usually deal with cancer." Why didn't I come back at her with something clever like, "Well I must be his first?" Instead I proceeded to tell her too much info by saying, "I have irregular cells which are a pre-cancerous condition and because I am a high risk patient, my insurance company and the doctors agree, I need to get my second breast removed." She said, "Well you do not have cancer so I cannot send this information to the local support group." I said, "I did have cancer in my other breast." She ignored me and asked if I had any other health issues. How could a trained "nurse" who sees many people every day with many health problems treat me like this? More importantly is why did I put up with it? I left the hospital hurt and discouraged. Was she just cold and uncaring? Did she treat everyone like this? I guess I will never know the answer to those questions. Should I have been like my friend and said, "I am older than 50 and I am not going to put up with people like you." If I would have been vocal and said those words it would have been an interesting turn of events. I am not sure it would have done me a bit of good because the nurse had decided I did not have breast cancer and I should not be having my breast removed. She acted like I had made the choice of having my breast removed for a trivial reason. I would think a nurse would know better. I just do not think she cared, I was just a piece of paper to her and my feelings did not matter one way or the other. I know being around her did not make me feel any better about myself. She could have been what caused a deep depression to take over my thoughts. I kept thinking I was not going to make it through this surgery. I did not tell anyone. I kept telling myself, "Stop being a drama queen, you are not going to die." In spite of the pep talks I gave myself in my mind I prepared for the possibility of death.

I threw a Mother's Day Tea a week before Mother's Day. The closer it came to having the tea I began to think, "This is my goodbye Tea." I had it in my mind the people who showed up really cared about me and the ones who did not show up did not care. It may be very unfair but it is how I felt. Only a few people knew I was having surgery at the end of the month because I had decided to wait till after surgery this time to tell most people. I felt the Tea Party I was throwing would let me know who wanted to see me. Two of my friends were sick and could not come. One friend lives in out of state and could not attend but she did send me a Mother's Day card and a Tea book full of recipes. I did feel these people cared about me, even though they could not attend my Tea. I had a wonderful time at the Tea. My youngest daughter Jessie came and helped me set up the Tea and she brought my grandson who was a joy at the Tea, he was the center of attention.

The friends who attended the Tea were Jean, Paula, Dessie and her daughter-in-law. They did not know how much it meant to me that they had attended my Tea. When someone is faced with a life and death situation the people who care about them need to call, write and visit. When someone is facing surgery they need to know the people whom they love and care about feel the same way. It was good to know the people who came to my Tea did it because they cared about seeing me and wanted to spend time with me. It was great to have the Tea to get my mind off of my upcoming surgery.

To keep busy the days before my surgery I cooked. Cooking relived my stress and kept my mind occupied. I baked like a mad woman: chocolate covered strawberry cake, bourbon cheesecake, and rhubarb/strawberry upside down cake. I invited my friend Jean to come over and share the bourbon cheesecake because she and her husband were bourbon enthusiasts. She sat with me and talked for two hours. Her husband had been diagnosed with bladder cancer in stage four, ten years ago and had survived after having chemo and radiation, so she could relate to my surgery anxiety. It was so good to talk to someone who could relate. But I still could not shake the negative thoughts in my head that I was not going to make it through this surgery.

The day of my surgery I sent my mom a picture of some flowers I had placed on my father's grave. It is a long and confusing story: my mom does not get to see my Dads grave because she lives in Florida and he did also when he died however he always told her," When I die bury me in Ohio," because it is where he lived most of his life. He requested to be buried in Ohio so that is where my mother buried him. Because of this she never gets to see his grave so she always asks me if I have gone to my dad's grave to put flowers on it. I knew the picture of his grave with flowers decorating it would make her feel good. I sent my oldest daughter Shawndra an article and a note about craft beer (she loves craft beers) and I mailed both letters to them on the way to surgery. I had been with my youngest and my grandson a lot before my surgery and I felt I had let them know how much I loved them. I had been getting along great with my husband so I know he knew how much I loved him. I felt I had done everything I could to connect with the people I loved just in case I did pass away during surgery.

The second surgery went well and my plastic surgeon did an amazing job. I was thankful I woke up after surgery and I prayed and thanked God he had saved me to live another day. I did not beat myself up for thinking prior to surgery I was not going to wake up. I just rejoiced in the fact I survived the surgery. I think a quote I recently saw on the TV show Political Animals applies here: "Most of life is hard it is filled with failure and loss, people disappoint you, dreams do not work out, hearts get broken, innocent people die, and the best moments of life when everything comes together are few however you'll never get to the next great moment if you do not keep going, so that's what I do . . . I keep going." I am glad God saw fit to let me keep going so I can get to the next great moment. I was thankful because I survived the surgery but my chest looked like a battleground.

Mastectomy Number Two vs. Number One

*I*MMEDIATELY AFTER MY second mastectomy I noticed something different. I started comparing the first mastectomy with the second mastectomy. A very glaring difference was I did not have bruises all over in odd places. With the first surgery I had bruises under my arms, on my hips and on my belly. The general surgeon who performed the first surgery even commented at my first office visit after the surgery, "Do you bruise easily because you have a lot of bruises." It just makes me think that I was not handled carefully during the first surgery. The male nurse at my second mastectomy said he would watch over me and make sure I was taken good care of. The plastic surgeon had forgotten to order the anti-nausea medicine put in my IV so instead they were going to have to inject it in my hand. I was proud of myself because both the plastic surgeon and the anesthesiologist tried to tell me I did not need the anti-nausea medicine but I insisted that they give it to me. They had made a mistake so they tried to cover it up by telling me I did not need the drug. I stood up for myself because I did not want to become constipated and deathly sick to my stomach after my surgery.

That is what happened to me after my first mastectomy and I was not going to go through that experience again without a fight. My male nurse tried to distract me while they did the injection by showing me the tattoos on his forearms. He even held my hand while they injected the anti-nausea medicine into my left hand, which was a surprisingly painful injection. His tattoos were quite fascinating. He had one on each arm of his two children's baby feet and their birth dates. He also came and checked on me after my surgery while I was still unconscious. My husband said he peeked in the recovery room and said, "I told her I would take care of her and I did." I tell everyone he was my nurse angel. What this wonderful nurse did reminds me of a quote from Martha N. Beck, "Angels come in many shapes and sizes, and most of them are not invisible."

So I guess the reason why I had all those bruises with my first surgery and not my second was because I did not have a nurse "angel" protecting me at my first mastectomy. I believe anyone getting surgery should be treated gently and with kindness while they are unconscious. I believe it is the surgeon's job to make sure their patient is taken care of. The general surgeon at my first surgery did not make sure I was taken good care of.

Another thing I noticed that was very different was the level of pain. I wondered, "Why was the pain so much worse after my first surgery and why did the pain last so much longer after the first surgery than after my second surgery? After my first surgery I passed out from the pain while I was at home trying to move from one couch to another. The pain was horrible. After the second surgery the pain was not nearly as bad. I could move from one couch to the other and get up and use the bathroom without passing out or feeling like my stitches were ripping open. After my first surgery I went to bed and stayed there for a couple days because every time I tried to sit in a chair I felt like my chest was ripping open. Could the way a surgeon cut me during my mastectomy make so much of a difference? Well in my case the hands of a plastic surgeon sure made a big difference in the way my surgery turned out. After my second surgery I felt better because I was not in so much pain. Visually the scars were less severe and healed faster with less pain involved.

Also with my first surgery I asked my doctor if he could give me something for post-surgery nausea in my IV. He said it was normal to get sick after surgery and I could take over the counter anti-nausea meds when I got home. Well his advice did not work and I stayed sick for two weeks. During those two weeks I became constipated and by the fourth day because I had not had a bowel movement I was hurting so bad when I sat down sharp pains shot up my back. The constipation was very severe and hurt so much. I finally just started walking around the house singing and crying. I think my husband thought I was losing my mind. With my second mastectomy I told my doctor about how sick I get after anesthesia and he had the anesthesiologist give me an anti-nausea shot prior to my surgery. When I got home I was not sick for two weeks and I was not constipated for four days. I wonder why my general surgeon ignored my request for anti-nausea medicine. Why would a doctor not give a patient something which would make them feel better once they got home?

I know one thing would have made me feel better after my first surgery: drainage tubes which actually worked correctly. When I got home from my first mastectomy surgery I noticed one tube was not working. When I saw the doctor the first week and told him the drain was not working he pulled it out (a very painful process when he did it) and put in another one. When I got home the tube he had just put in did not work and the second drain quit working during that week also. When I saw him the third week he removed both drains. When he removed the tubes old blood poured all over the table and onto the floor and my clothes. The blood had backed up because the drains did not work properly. The smell was awful and the amount of dark red almost black colored blood which came out was shocking. At the time I knew something was not right. I now know this kind of thing does not have to happen because my drainage tube worked fine after my second mastectomy. My plastic surgeon told me that drains that become clogged, result in retained fluid that can contribute to infection or other complications. Drains that did not work could have attributed to the reason why I remained sick so long after my first mastectomy.

After my second mastectomy my doctor put in only one drain and it worked for five days. I saw him at his office and he took it out gently (no pain involved) and said it had done its job. He said he could tell because the color of the blood draining was no longer red instead it was a yellowish color which meant I did not need any more draining done to my wound. If you have ever had a drainage tube put in after surgery you know what a big relief it is to get it removed after five days. The drainage tube is put in through a hole which is cut out during surgery. Then the tube is inserted in the hole and attached via a couple stitches. The tube is then taped to the patient's stomach. It is a long dangly plastic tube which the blood from a person's surgery drains into. At the end of the tube is a sealed cup. The cup has to be opened and drained a couple times a day after surgery. It smells bad, it is hard to take a shower and it is hard to cover up when a person goes out in public. I stuffed mine in my bra and wore loose clothes. After my first surgery I had to put up with not one but two drains which did not work, were not taken out till the second week and once they were taken out left a bucket of blood gushing out because they did not work correctly. At the time it made me furious and it also makes me furious to think about it now.

I was so glad the second time around none of those horrible things happened. I did my own research and opted for a plastic surgeon to perform my second surgery. Because of my research I did not have to go through the pain and suffering I had experienced during and after my first surgery! It makes me sad to think about all the unnecessary pain I went through. I feel blessed the second time around. I found a wonderful doctor who saved me from all the pain. The bonus of the second mastectomy was I also had an angel nurse with the baby footprint tattoos on his arms that helped me through the fear I felt in the operating room prior to my surgery.

The healing time from my second surgery was nothing compared to my first. I am glad I have both mastectomies over with and I can have some peace of mind. Unfortunately my silicone implants do not match. The plastic surgeon told me I am going to have to get one final surgery. The general surgeon left a straight long scar when he did my first mastectomy and the plastic surgeon left a upside down "T" shaped scar after he did my second mastectomy. He said he wants to do another surgery because he thinks he can go in and adjust the first silicone implant to make it look more like the new implant. Because the scars left my breasts shaped so differently it is hard for my plastic surgeon to get the silicone implants to look identical. I decided to think about it before I make any decisions about additional surgeries. I realize how lucky I am to be alive but the previous surgeries have left me with a mild case of IBS. My MD said the IBS is my body's reaction to the anesthesia I received during each surgery. I am not sure I can psych myself up for another surgery on my breasts. I found a quote from the Cancer Reconstruction—PRMA Plastic Surgery, San Antonio, TX website which describes how I feel about my breasts, "Every scar I have makes me who I am."

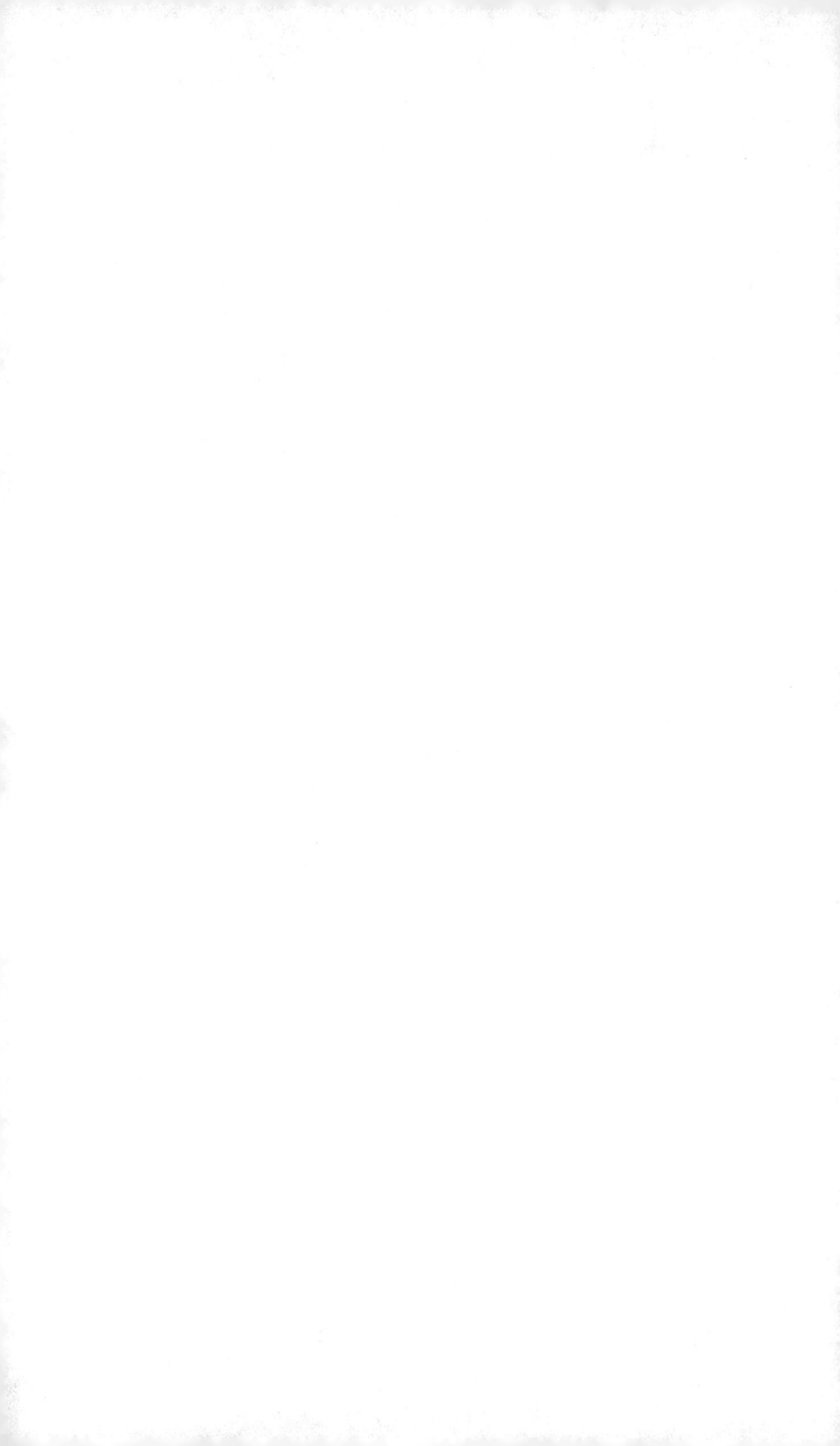

Perfect Breasts

I AM STILL recovering physically and mentally from two mastectomies in just two years. I had an implant put in both sides so my chest is not flat. My implant breasts are nipple free and they do not have the same sensitivity to touch that my real breasts did. On my right breast I had one surgery: a mastectomy with a silicone implant put in at the same time. My left breast had Stage zero duct cancer so they could not put in a silicone implant while they performed the mastectomy because they thought I may have to have chemo or radiation. My left breast had four reconstruction surgeries and with each surgery the same scar was opened then stitched closed. Because of the numerous surgeries this scar is deep and thick. In a two year period I had five breast surgeries, two biopsy surgeries, four saline injections (which made me sick for a week each time and was so painful I felt like I had gotten another surgery) two MRI's and four mammograms.

Now that the painful surgeries were over I began to ask myself why me? Why did I get breast cancer? What did I do wrong? Did I get too fat? Did I eat too much chocolate? Did I use the wrong deodorant? This feeling of guilt has been made ten times worse by the thoughtless comments of other people when I tell them about my breast cancer. When I told a relative about my second mastectomy and about the "lesions" and or "irregular cells" (doctor jargon) she acted like I had not even said anything and instead proceeded to tell me about her upcoming possible surgery and a family member's "self-diagnosis" of Cancer." Which I am positive is not a disease one can diagnose themselves. It was an odd and uncaring reaction, especially from a family member. I also wondered, "When did news about cancer become a competition about who is the sickest person in the family?" What did I expect? When I told her about the cancer in my first breast two years ago, these were her comments: "Are you sure? Did you misunderstand the doctor? Are you over reacting? The Dr. probably meant something else?" Then she proceeded to tell me about all the people she knew who had their breasts removed and it was "As easy as pie." When I told another family member about my first breast cancer diagnosis, she proceeded to tell me I had used the wrong deodorants, taken the wrong medicine and gained too much weight over the years. My youngest sister had a friend who said she heard from a friend, breast reductions (something I had gotten two years before my first mastectomy) caused breast cancer. I got the message loud and clear. These people were blaming me for my cancer. Wow they could not be more mean and thoughtless.

Why do women act this way and say the awful things they say to women with breast cancer? Is it because they are secretly thinking, "thank god it is you not me?" Or "She deserves it for X number of reasons" or are they just at a loss for words? Either way it hurts to be treated like a person that has something contagious or to be subjected to rude and thoughtless comments. Careless comments flung at someone when they are too stunned to respond, are sometimes unforgiveable. I found a site on Facebook which explains exactly what I am talking about, "Words which stab anyone with a chronic illness like a knife to the heart":

- Maybe you could exercise and lose a little weight?
- You do not look sick.

- My Aunt had the same thing you have and now she is fine.
- Maybe you just need some rest?
- There is a supplement you can take which can cure your condition.
- Maybe you just need to get out of the house more?

All of the above "stabs" have been aimed, by various people, at my heart since this crazy journey began. The sad thing is most people do not know or do not care about the words they have thoughtlessly spouted out of their mouths. They do not think twice about the deep wounds they have inflicted into the soul of an already wounded cancer victim. When someone is sick they blame themselves. They ask themselves if getting cancer was their fault. People who are sick do not need questions or "advice" from others. Cancer patients are always running an internal battery of questions in their head. One of the questions I asked myself was: "Did I do everything I should have to prevent getting cancer?" To answer my own questions I went over the list of things researchers have said to do to help prevent breast cancer. I wanted to see if I had done the things researchers have suggested a woman do to prevent breast cancer. I had gotten regular mammograms, I gave birth to two children and breast fed them and I had always done some form of exercise. These are the things researchers suggest a woman do to help prevent breast cancer. Ok I had followed the guideline researchers suggest are breast cancer preventers so why did I still get cancer?

Maybe as my sister's friend suggested I got cancer because I had previously gotten breast reduction surgery. I wanted to know the answer so I did research on breast reductions and studies show breast reductions do not cause breast cancer. Research shows having breast reductions actually help some women because the person who reads the mammogram has less tissue to look at so results are clearer. I also looked at the possibility of using the "wrong" deodorant to see if it was a cause of my breast cancer. A relative suggested that using the wrong deodorant could be the reason why I got cancer. I read that the American Cancer Society finds no clear link between deodorant/antiperspirants and breast cancer. In a posting on the American Cancer Society Web page they note, "There are no strong epidemiological studies in the medical literature which link breast cancer risk and antiperspirant use, and there is very little scientific evidence to support this claim."

I wondered did I get breast cancer because during the last 12 years I had put on some extra pounds. Was it my weakness for chocolate? I looked at the research on eating "too much chocolate" (which I personally do not believe is "humanly possible to do" which was probably the philosophy that caused my weight gain in the first place) to see if this could be a cause of breast cancer. I did not find anything linking the consuming of chocolate to breast cancer. A lot of research does suggest if a person eats small amounts of chocolate it is actually good for their heart. It may help lower blood pressure and can help the brain function better. This was news which the chocolate lover in my soul embraced wholeheartedly. Last but not least I also looked into weight gain and how it related to breast cancer and found this information: (from the Cancer Research Journal): "Our findings support weight loss through calorie reduction and increased exercise as a means for reducing inflammatory biomarkers and thereby potentially reducing cancer risk in overweight and obese postmenopausal women," said researchers led by Dr. Anne McTiernan, director of the Prevention Center at the Fred Hutchinson Cancer Research Center, in Seattle. So according to this info becoming overweight in the past 12 years was the reason I got breast cancer?

This theory did not make a lot of sense because many women I know are overweight or obese and they do not have breast cancer. Also many skinny women get breast cancer. So if breast reductions, eating chocolate and using the "wrong" deodorant did not "cause my cancer" what did cause my cancer? Should I believe that my weight gain caused it? If so was it my fault that I got cancer? J. Johnson said, "I think there comes a point when a person must stop beating themselves up over mistakes they made in the past.

The mistakes someone made in the past should be left in the past. Little do we realize nobody is perfect?" As a matter of fact, life just would not be any fun if we were perfect, (this is a theory I hold on to tightly to because I know I will never be perfect) there would be no room for growth, and we would live our lives with no direction and no purpose. I had one purpose to find out why I got breast cancer. I wondered, "Did I get breast cancer because of the genes I inherited?"

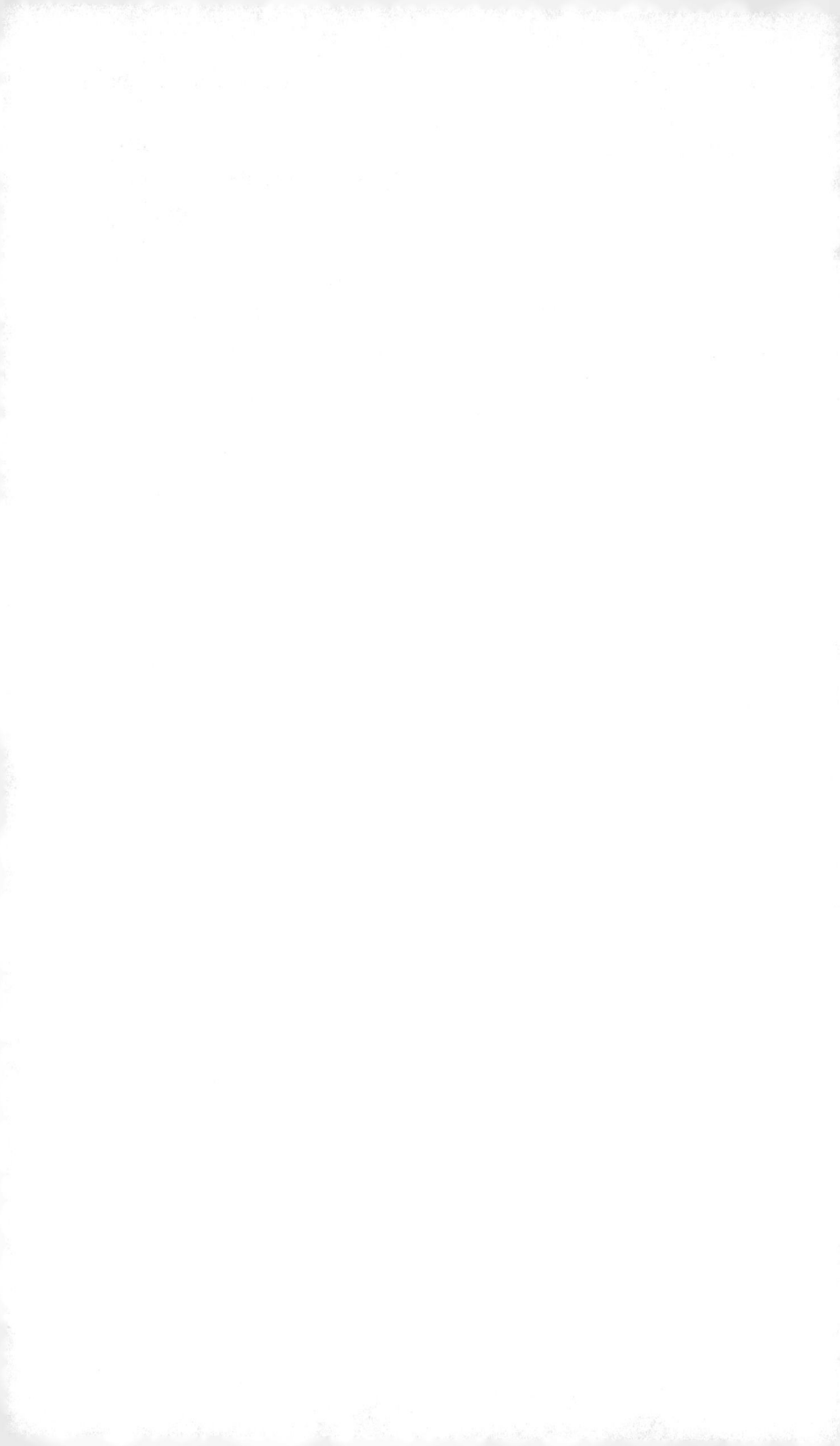

An Adopted Child

HE FIRST QUESTION the doctors always asked about my breast cancer is, "Does breast cancer run in your family?" This question should be simple enough to answer for me it was not. I was adopted at the age of two and I have no recollection of any other life. Previously when I filled out family medical history on any questionnaire form at the doctor's office, I used my adopted mom and dad's history without thinking. It did not cross my mind that my adopted parent's medical history did not reflect my medical history. Now that I had breast cancer I knew I had to find out more about my real family history. My adoption was a family adoption, meaning if my adopted mother had not adopted me she would be my aunt. The story I have always been told about my adoption, by my adopted mother and my blood grandmother is this: my aunt's (my adopted mother) younger brother Bob and his wife, Kaye were having marital problems. They left me with my grandmother a lot and when they left me with her I was always hungry and had a wet diaper. I also had a lot of nightmares and my grandmother was very concerned. She knew Kaye and Bob were fighting a lot and she was afraid the fights were the cause of my nightmares. One time my aunt came over to visit my grandmother after I had been dropped off. I had been at my grandmother's house for over a week without any word from my parents. When my aunt and her family came over I cried to go home with them. She had four kids and she said I loved all the noise and commotion her big family made. My grandmother's house was quiet because only she and my grandfather lived there, and my grandfather was gone a lot of the time. They took me home with them and I never went back to live with my grandmother. My aunt informed me that my grandmother cried for weeks after I left. My "aunt" was afraid if she did not adopt me I may be put in foster care. So she and her husband started the adoption proceedings and I became part of their family. I guess Kaye and Bob were separated by then and neither one of them put up any resistance concerning my adoption. I always wondered why they gave me up for adoption. That question may never get answered because my birth mother passed away and my birth father is not in contact with the family. When I had my children I knew I could never give them up. They were not perfect children they did cry and they did have temper tantrums. I loved them so much and could not imagine life without them. Love is so important in life giving and receiving love is what life is all about. A Wise physician said, "The best medicine for humans is love. Someone asked, "If it does not work?" He smiled and answered, "I increase the dose," Wisdom quotes.

But my biggest concern now was not what had happened to me as a child it was finding out about my family health history. The reason I could not find out much about my family history is because a couple years after my adoption Kaye lost contact with the family and we did not hear from her. My mother did not talk about her and did not even tell me I was adopted until I was 11 years old. When I asked about Kaye's background my adopted mother knew very little. By the time I had been diagnosed with breast cancer my birth mother had died of congestive heart failure. My half-brother, Stevie called to tell me about her poor health a few months before she died. It was nice to be in contact with someone who had grown up with my birth mother and the bonus was I got to know a missing sibling. Someone I had never known. He had a different father than I did and he moved in with his father when he was 12. He explained how he was getting into a lot of trouble in school when he lived with our birth mother so his father took him in and he said it saved him. He said he loved living with his father and his step mom. He also started liking school and not getting into trouble at his new school. We talked a lot on the phone and on Facebook and once I found out I had breast cancer he was the one I asked about the history of breast cancer in Kaye's family. He said Kaye's mother had died of complications from compacted bowels and this was the only family health history he really knew about. He said Kaye only had brothers and they were never interested in getting to know him. I also have a younger sister, Gail, who lived with Kaye all her life. She found me on Facebook a year or so after my birth mother's death so when I found out about my cancer I asked her if she had ever had breast cancer. She said she had not. She also said she went regularly for breast exams and mammograms. She did not know anyone in the family who had breast cancer.

Breast cancer did not show up on my maternal side how about my paternal side? My father's (Bob) side was easy to trace because my adopted mother was Bob's sister. My grandmother was the same because she was their mother. She and her family had no history of breast cancer. So it appeared my cancer was not due to heredity. That was good to know because it meant my daughters would have less to worry about regarding breast cancer. They would not have to take the BRAC1 test that has been in the news lately. BRAC1 is a genetic test to see if you have inherited genes which make you predisposed to breast and ovarian cancer. Angelina Jolie has made this test famous because she let the public know that she had this test done because her aunt and mother both died from breast cancer. She wanted to see if she was genetically predisposed and from the test results she found that she was. She decided to have a double mastectomy and is considering having her ovaries removed. I appreciate what she has done because it makes me and other women like me feel less like freaks. If she can do it and still be a sex symbol then regular women can feel good about themselves also.

The Answer

*U*NLIKE ANGELIA I was not genetically predisposed to develop breast cancer. I decided to continue doing research to try to find out why I got breast cancer. I remembered something my GYN had told me in the past. He had referred to my breasts as "dense breasts." So I did research on this type of breast. A dense breast contributes to a higher risk factor. Research says that breast cancer is not formed in the fatty part of the breast. It is formed in the dense part of the breast. So the denser the breast the less fat it contains and the higher the chance I had to develop cancer. When I looked up the term dense breasts on the internet I found this information: dense breasts are a specific genetic condition which affects about one in six women. It's a characteristic, as well as a genetic condition. There's a huge range in breast density among women, with some exhibiting nearly all fat tissue in their breasts, while others have nearly none. If you go to the far end of the scale, to women with extremely dense breasts, recent studies have shown these women have about a four to six-time greater risk of breast cancer as women whose breasts are not dense. Scientists are not yet sure why this is, beyond the fact that cancer occurs in breast tissue, not fat; so the higher your ratio of breast tissue, the more opportunity you have to get breast cancer. So this was most likely the reason I developed breast cancer because my breasts were dense. I was satisfied with this answer and now I just needed to recover from all my surgeries and move on with my life.

Please Be Quiet About Your Cancer

I HAD LUNCH with a group of female friends. I began telling them about the bruises I had all over my body after my first mastectomy and I pondered out loud, "I wonder if I was not moved carefully or if the people at the hospital moved me around like a shack of feed. Was this the reason why I had so many bruises after my first surgery? What is even stranger is after my second surgery I had no bruises." My friend interrupted and said, "You need to forget all about your surgery problems because it was in the past and what is in the past needs to stay there." I think she was trying to make me stop talking about my bad experience because she is from the school of thought, "Pretend it did not happen and it did not." Or maybe she just did not want me to bring everyone down. I know from experience that talking about my cancer tends to bring everyone down and make them uncomfortable. I am trying to do what Lifehouse sings about, "I'm trying to find my way the best way that I know how." This is exactly what I am trying to do when I reminisce about the past I am trying to find my way to the future, the best way I know how.

I believe people do not learn life lessons if they forget about the past. If the movie stars I mentioned previously had hid their breast cancer I would not have read their stories and been inspired by them. I know my friend had the best of intentions I do not agree with her logic. I am glad my friend made that comment because it made me think about all the things we keep to ourselves. Her philosophy is if we do not think about our problems then they are in the past and we are over the hurt and pain. She believes it will be like the problems never happened. Ignoring my problems does not work for me. I do not believe it works for most people. I need to talk about the problems I had with my doctors. If my experiences were bad and if I feel I have been treated badly I need to talk about it. It makes me feel better to share my feelings about issues which concern me and when I do I usually get some insights into other people's experiences. It also helps me deal with my own problems. I discover how other people handle similar situations. I wondered if the simple truth was my friend really just did not want to hear about my cancer.

Even though my friend basically said what is past is forgotten, she proceeded to tell us about a doctor who had a terrible reputation in her town and how she went to him once in the past and has avoided going to him since that one visit. Another friend who was at lunch knew the doctor because they both grew up in the same town. She immediately started talking about how bad this particular doctor was and said, "I did not go to his office more than once because when I asked him questions he blew me off." I chimed in and shared my experience about the first doctor I went to when I discovered I was pregnant with my first child. I told my friends about how I tried to ask my doctor questions since it was my first experience with childbirth and instead of answering me the doctor said, "Here is a brochure read it." I was 24 and old enough to know a doctor should not treat a first time mother this way. I told them I went home and called another doctor and made an appointment. I then called the doctor I had just had an appointment with and told his receptionist. "I want to let you know I will not be seeing Dr. "Smith" again because as a first time mother I want a doctor who will answer my questions." My friends laughed and said they could relate to my experience. When I had questions about the information I had received from various doctors and medical staff it would have been encouraging for me to hear from friends who had similar problems. I know after I had all my surgeries it was encouraging to read about how other people had gone through the same experiences and came through it in still sane and in one piece. When someone finds out other people have similar problems they do not feel so alone. When I had my surgeries I needed all the encouragement I could get. That is why it felt so good to talk to other female friends about my cancer journey. Women do need each other and we are happier when we know we have a good female friend, relative, mother or daughter whom we can turn to in happy times and in sad times or someone we can just invite over for cheesecake and some gossip. It is good for our health and it is good for our soul.

History With my Female Friends

I WISH I would have made friendships with women a higher priority when I was younger. I did have friends and I loved to go to my friend's homes because it was fun to get out of my house. Most of my girlfriends had much more lenient parents than I had. Well at least the friend's houses I liked to go to did. Some of my friends had very strict parents. Going to their houses was not a lot of fun. The problem with going to my friend's houses was my mom did not like me to go. I had the feeling she did not trust me. She probably was just trying to keep me safe but at the time I felt like I was in a cage. She tried to prevent me from going to my friend's houses at every possible turn. When I did go I had a strict curfew. She usually would not let me stay with my friends at all if they had brothers. She said something bad might happen to me since there were boys in the house. She felt that boys and men could not control themselves around females.

I did manage to have at least one friend at all times throughout my school years and they wanted to be my friend in spite of everything. When I turned 16 I was allowed to go on double dates with my girlfriends and their boyfriends. Double dating worked out well for a while however when my boyfriend and I became serious he really did not like to go out with other couples. I dropped my friends and graduated from high school one year early. I moved to a town close by and lived with my grandmother. I got a fast food job so I could have my own money. Living with my grandmother was wonderful because she trusted me and was not always keeping track of me or grounding me. I was only seventeen but I felt like I was much older than that. A year later I got married and devoted myself to my marriage and a few years later to my daughters. My husband was always telling me jokes and making me laugh so I thought of him as a good friend. We went to our family's houses for holidays and we occasionally double dated with friends. I never had a close girlfriend during those times. I remember feeling very lonely before I had kids because my husband worked seven days a week so I was alone a lot. I did not try to make friends because he did not like people over and he liked me to be there when he came home from work. Once my daughters were born I just kept myself busy and did not try and make friends. As my daughters grew I loved going places with them and laughing and having fun with them and their friends. I was a girl scout leader, I shuttled other peoples kids to various events and I even sat with other mothers at various school and sporting events however I did not have a girlfriend to just hang out with for many years.

A woman who I was a friend of mine when I was in elementary school and in high school lived close and had a son the same age as my daughter Jessie. She and I began spending a lot of time together. Sometimes taking our kids with us or just going out in a group with other ladies. We also did couple things with our husbands and other couples. I really liked having a girlfriend again. My husband did not like going places with other couples so I quit trying to set up double dates with my friend and her husband. Instead she and I began taking our kids to movies, skating and to local amusement parks. We had some great times together. She began working with a lady who did not like me and I pulled away from our friendship because she insisted on inviting this lady to everything we did together. Even though we were not as close as we previously had been she did help me find a job. She told her sister that I was looking for work and her sister got a job for me working part-time at the College where she was employed. I worked with the sister for a while. After I worked for the College part-time for one year I got a full-time job with the same College in another department. For a while I only ate lunch with her sister because I felt we had become good friends while I worked in her department. Slowly I began making girlfriends in my new office and going to lunch with them instead.

When I began working full time I was so exhausted by the end of the work week I really did not care if I was a couch potato the entire weekend. The friends I made at work were just work friends. We went out to lunch however I did not see them any other time outside of work. My friend's sister and I would get together with another lady she knew once a month. We also made sure to celebrate birthdays together. We also took a girlfriend trip to Las Vegas. When I quit my job and my husband and I opened a sandwich shop in the little college town where I previously worked, I was overwhelmed with running a business and very stressed out most of the time. I was working seven days a week and had little time for girlfriends. When I had been running the sandwich shop for six months I started cutting back on my hours. This freed up some of my time. The three of us started getting together again once a month. For some reason I really did not enjoy our ladies nights. Maybe I felt like they were jealous because I owned my own business? They both always talked about how much they would like to have a business of their own. Sometimes they made "funny" comments which I thought were snide. Saying things like, "Why did you hire a person who everyone knows is a loser," and other comments like, "I bet you wish you were back at your old job." They wanted to meet in December to exchange Christmas gifts but I keep telling them I was too busy to see them. I made these excuses because the last few times we had been together I did not enjoy myself. When we finally did see each other in February to celebrate my birthday, I shared a problem with them that I was having with my daughter. In so many words they both basically told me I was a terrible mother. Maybe in their opinion I was being a terrible mother. I felt good friends would have given me the benefit of the doubt or at least spoken some comforting words to encourage me. I had laid my heart out on the line and they had proceeded to kick me when I was down. I did not feel like good friends would treat me in such a manner and I had not felt like they had been good friends for quite a while. I went home and wrote them an email telling them just how I felt and that I needed a break from them. I never heard back from either one of them so I guess I was right we were not good friends. I now realize the level of stress I was under running my own business probably factored into the end of our friendships. Since I started the restaurant my top two priorities were my business and my family.

I did not get to see my work friends at work anymore and no longer shared lunches with them. So when I did get to see them I really enjoyed spending time with them. I realized how much I missed them. We began meeting for dinners or weekend lunches when we had time. I owned my own business and employed young college students. I really missed working with women my age. I began cherishing my time with other women and I cherished my female friends more. It was good to get together with other women and talk about the unique issues women go through. It is fun to talk with my girlfriends about our past. Things which use to crush us we can now share with each other and laugh about it. One story I recently shared with my friends was a story about how as junior high student I was constantly being accused of stuffing my bra. I always felt hurt and embarrassed. Life did a 360 and it became necessary to stuff my bra because one side of my chest was flat after my first surgery. So if someone were to yell at me after my first surgery, "She is wearing falsies" like the mean boys did back in Junior High, they would have been half right. I am glad I can laugh about something which happened to me in sixth grade.

Something that back then I thought was the "end of the world." I now realize it was a life lesson.

Hanging out with girlfriends is such a wonderful thing for women to do. We can relate to each other and share our ups and downs. We do not have to leave it in the past and not talk about it like my friend suggested. We can share our problems. We do not have to feel that we need to hide bad things that happen in our lives. We share our souls and even when we disagree with each other we can still learn something. I continue to find new female friends the more I socialize or do volunteer work. I made a couple of friends by volunteering at a local political office and other friends by joining an on-line Meetup group. I also enjoy doing things with my daughters. My daughter Jessie and I see each other a lot because she lives near me. When my youngest and I get together we always laugh and have fun. We find the same things funny and have a lot in common. My oldest daughter, Shawndra lives 14 hours away so I do not get to see her much. When I do see her we always have a good time. She is busy doing about 10 freelance jobs and she and her husband have tons of friends and a busy social life. I went with her recently to San Francisco to attend a couple of private winery tours. She was sent there by one of her clients to write about two small wineries. We had fun and explored the city. She is so full of life and loves life, being with her is always a pleasure.

Jean, a good friend of mine found an essay talking about how important our female friends and relatives are to our health. After having breast cancer I am always searching for ways to improve my health. So if being with friends and sharing my experiences is good for my health that is what I will continue to do. The essay said one of the best things a man can do for his heath is to be married and one of the best things a woman can do for her health is to nurture her relationships with other women. It went on to say how women feel connected with each other in a different way than the way we connect with men. It also talked about how we provide support systems and how we help each other deal with stress and difficult life experiences. The essay said research also shows how physically this quality "girlfriend time" helps us to create more serotonin which helps us combat depression and create a general feeling of well-being.

In the article, <u>Why Friendships Are So Important</u>, by Sheryl Kraft, she quotes Aristotle who said: "Without friends no one would choose to live, though he had all other goods." Studies show that women bond by sharing their feelings while men bond by doing activities together. When women share our feelings we also share our souls. For us spending time with a friend is as important as jogging or working out at the gym. When we exercise we are doing great things for our bodies. But sometimes we feel when we are having fun with other women; we are wasting our time and should be doing more productive things. We need to stop feeling guilty about spending fun quality time with other females. We need to realize friendships with our girlfriends, mothers, sisters and daughters are very good for both our mental and physical health.

Great Doctors

I KNOW SEEING a good doctor was much better for my mental health than seeing a bad doctor. I have had some great doctors. One of those great doctors was my GYN. He was great from the very beginning. He called in person to tell me the bad news about my breast cancer something all doctors, I later discovered, do not do. He did send me to a general surgeon who I ended up not liking. However I do not blame him for recommending someone he thought was a good doctor. I think he really believed in the surgeon who he recommended. Unfortunately the general surgeon he recommended did not have the bedside manner or the kind and caring nature it takes to perform mastectomies. Even though the general surgeon should have never performed my first surgery I did like a couple things about him prior to my surgery. He gave me his cell phone number and said to call him anytime. He thought my husband and I were "too emotional" and I think he was afraid without the hope of calling him we may just fall apart. He also prescribed one week of sleeping pills when I told him I could not sleep. So even though I would never recommend him to perform a mastectomy on anyone, I did appreciate those two things he did. If we do not find the good things in life I think we would all just lose our minds due to all the negativity which surrounds us.

One negative thing I am still dealing with is the conflicting information I still get from various doctors. I am confused about a piece of information I was given after my first surgery versus my second surgery. I was told after my first mastectomy I no longer needed to get a mammogram on the left side because the breast tissue was no longer there. After my second mastectomy I was told I needed to get mammograms and do self-checks with my breasts. I have been doing research on the internet and a lot of doctors agree patients should get a baseline mammogram six months after their mastectomy surgery. So with all this conflicting information I will just have to ask my doctors if they will do a mammogram and if they will not I will have to find a doctor who does. I feel as a patient we are given so much information and when it is conflicting information we are confused and scared because we trust our doctors to tell us the correct information. After seeing so many doctors I really would not mind if I never had to see another doctor the rest of my life.

When my second biopsy was read differently by various doctors I told the office that performed my biopsy, "I am just the patient, I am not a doctor and all I can do is believe what the doctors tell me." It makes a patient feel very helpless to have to "be the doctor" by doing the work the doctor should have done. In my case I feel the oncologist should have followed through and had more tests done on my breast. I felt very vulnerable, scared and uncared for by her. I felt like I was not a real person. I was a piece of paper she decided she was done with. When I had my first surgery I did not get a double mastectomy because my doctor advised against it. I now realize I would have been best if I would have gotten a second opinion and I should have been sent to an oncologist before my surgery. I was following my surgeon's orders because I trusted him. I now know my trust was unfounded which makes me feel vulnerable, scared, and uncared for. Now I take charge of my healthcare. I do research on my own and get a second, third or fourth opinion before I take the word of one doctor. Because I was given conflicting information before, during and after my first surgery I am now a cautious and more informed patient and I hope if I have any future health problems I will do lots of research and get more than one opinion from one doctor. I feel like the bad experiences I have been though have made me a patient who will stand up for her rights. It has also made me a person who appreciates things she never did before.

I did not appreciate my big breasts when I had them. I took them for granted and thought of them as a nuisance. I got a breast reduction in 2009 not knowing just two years later I would have breast cancer. Just about the time my breast reduction surgery scars were fading and I felt like I was going to have normal breasts again, I found out I had breast cancer. Life is full of ironies. When I got my breast reduction I worried about how ugly the scars were, little did I know I was going to have mastectomy scars much more frightening than my reduction scars. Now that the second breast has been removed my chest looks like a battlefield of scars. The right side is not so bad because the plastic surgeon only had to preform one surgery on that side. In his line of work the appearance of the scars after the surgery are very important. My left breast has some ugly scars and lots of broken blood veins from when the saline injections were put in to stretch the skin. I may never have normal breasts again. I really did not appreciate the wonderful breasts I use to have. As they say sometimes you do not realize how good something is until it is gone. The most important lesson I have learned because of this experience is to appreciate the things I have and the people who love me.

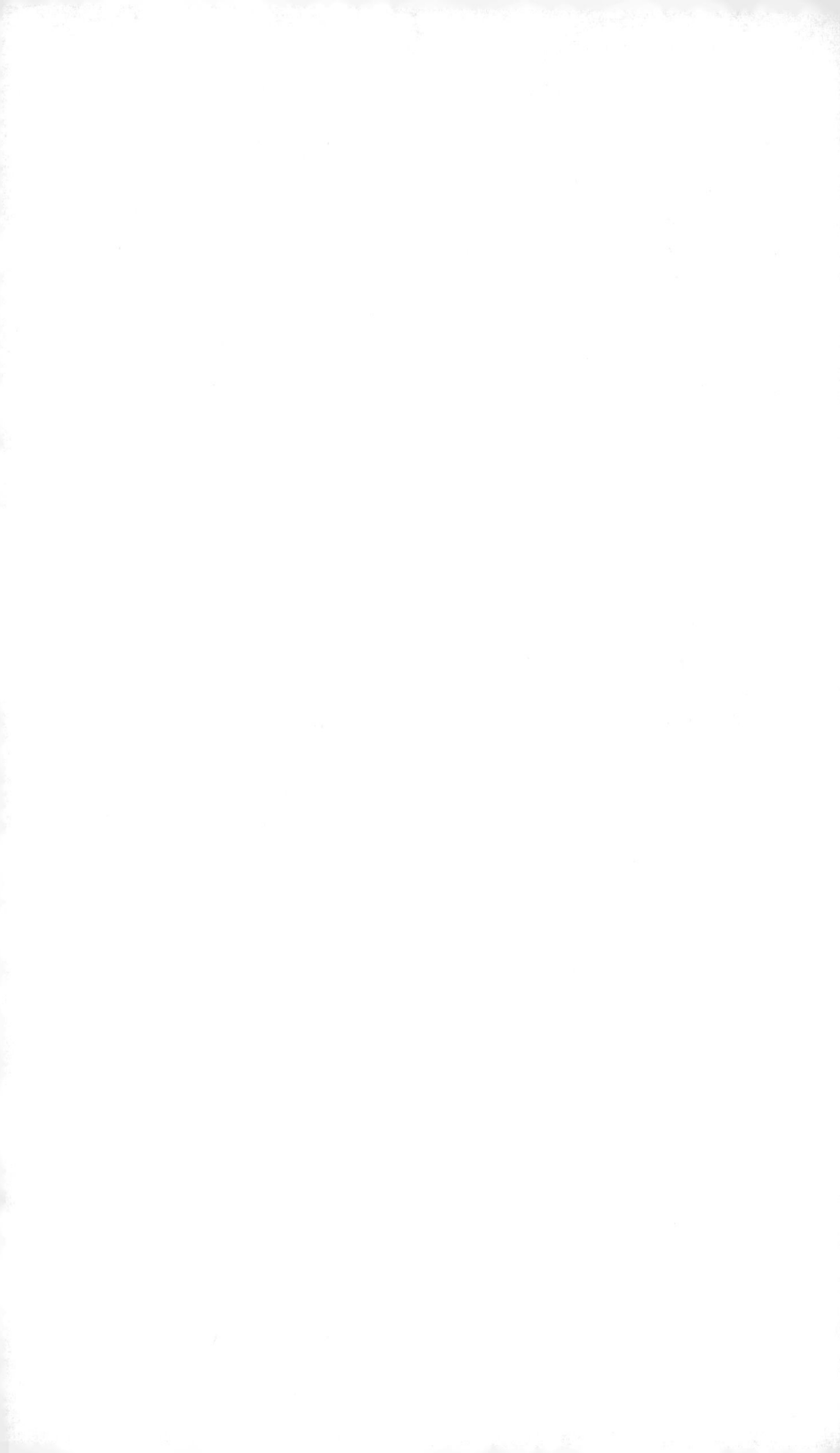

You Just Said What?

I AM LUCKY to have people love me but I also have had people say rude/dumb/crazy things to me about my cancer or my breasts on more than one occasion. I realize it was never my breasts or my cancer which were the problem it was the people who made horrible comments and my reaction to the things they said. What I would like to say to the next person who says something stupid about my cancer is repeat this quote which I found on Facebook, "Do not judge me; you cannot handle half of what I've dealt with. There are reasons I do the things I do, there are reasons I am who I am," (Anonymous). To my own amusement I assume the dumb people who say mean and rude things to me about my cancer would not be smart or deep enough to handle the depth of that quote. So when random people I meet in life say dumb things about breast cancer should I retaliate with a nasty comment?

What about people who I see on a regular basis? When it comes to friends and family: is it okay for them to say rude things because they may be nice the next time I see them? Should I say something rude back to strangers when they say careless things because I will never see them again? Should I let friends continue to make rude and thoughtless comments in the hope they will make up for it later? When my friend said she was tired of being nice because she was 50 now and had been nice all her life, it made me laugh and I could relate so much to what she was saying. It also made me realize I am not alone other women feel like they also have been treated rudely and have had crazy or mean things said to them. Just like me they usually just take it and do not respond with a nasty comeback of their own. Maybe I will become like my friend and be tired of being nice. Maybe I will give people back what they give when they are rude. Or maybe I will decide dumb and thoughtless people just are not worth my time and energy?

One of my relatives made a very dumb and thoughtless comment she said, "You wanted to get the surgery because you did not have faith the Lord would heal you." After my diagnosis, I have had far too many people treat my mastectomies as something I did not really need to get done. Something I wanted to get done out of fear.

Some people I knew acted like they did not agree with the decision that the doctors and I had made. They acted like I had chosen to have optional plastic surgery. During my first breast removal people would say things like, "Oh it was pre-cancer so you really did not have cancer!" Or, "Is Stage zero cancer even really cancer?" It never seemed like they were asking me a question. It seemed like these people were judging me. When my second breast was diagnosed as "irregular cells and lesions," some people thought I should not get my breast removed. I would tell these naysayers, "The doctors told me this condition has a high risk of becoming cancer." They disagreed with the doctors and thought I should wait to see if cancer did show up. It is hard to explain anything to people who think they know more than the doctors do. It is difficult to be around people who do not care enough to realize how hard it was for me to make the decision to have my breast removed. I have to get used to people being rude or naïve. I just have to know I made the right choice for me with some help from good doctors.

I recently decided one lady I know is not worth my time. I thought we were becoming friends so the first time she said something stupid/rude I let it slide. She said that if she ever was diagnosed with breast cancer she would not get a mastectomy because she would rather die than have her breasts removed. I told her that was her choice and I changed the subject. A couple of months later she sat at a restaurant eating dinner with me and a mutual acquaintance of ours. We were discussing wine and how it only takes one glass to get buzzed now that we are over 50. Somehow the conversation made her start talking about her how her breasts have changed since she turned 50. She said that her breasts use to be amazing and perky but now they were a little saggy. She then said that she asked her GYN about it and the GYN told her that in her opinion my "friend" had amazing breasts. So my "friend" said she guessed she would have to love her breasts now because they GYN had raved about them. She went on like this for at least 10 minutes. She chuckled and finally shut up. I sat there thinking what kind of a person would talk about her breasts not being as perky as they use to be then go on and on about her breasts pretending to complain about them in front of a woman that had two mastectomies? Maybe I was being too sensitive but my "friend" was being very insensitive. I think this "friend" was a test. As Judy Belmont (via Emotional Wellness for Positive Living) put it, "She reached a point in her life where she stopped valuing others that did not value her. In letting them go she was finally able to get herself back." I think I am going to let this "friend" go.

No matter what friends, family or foes say to me I have to live with myself and I have to decide if I want to come back with a witty or snide remark or if I want to just let it roll off my shoulders. I have never taken pleasure in returning an insult with an insult. I never feel good about myself when I do insult someone. I know I do not want to be like a relative of mine who walks around with a chip on her shoulder just waiting for people to do something she does not like. She constantly thinks people have said something mean or have bad intentions. It gives her a reason to be mad at the world. She is always so sure the world is out to get her. I really do not want to live my life that way. Is there a happy medium? With all I have been through are a few rude remarks about my breasts or anything else worth losing sleep over? I have to accept the way my breasts look now versus the way they use to look. Because I do not like to see people suffer no matter how much they make me suffer I think I will try and let rude or thoughtless comments roll off my shoulders. This quote says exactly how I feel: "The saddest people smile the brightest the most damaged people are the wisest. All because they do not wish to see anyone else suffer the way they do," Anonymous.

People Whom I Love

I READ THAT the average person has two or three people they can call friends. They defined a friend as someone you could count on to be by your side in bad times or good times. I was lucky that I had more than three people that I could call my friends during my cancer journey. They say a person finds their true friends and the people who really love them when they go through hard times and I agree with that. I am thankful for the people who stepped up to the plate and cared enough about me to help me though the pain. I just hope I will be there for them in the good times and especially in the bad times. What I continue to learn is people are surprising. The people that you assume will support you sometimes will not and the ones you do not expect to show any kind of support are there for you. I thank God for the people who helped me through my pain and suffering and for the people who have been kind during moments I least expected it. I had a nurse by the name of Mary at my first silicone implant surgery. She was also my prep nurse at the second mastectomy. She told me about her breast cancer experience. She said my plastic surgeon had done her silicone implant surgery when she had breast cancer and he was so good to her. She said she would recommend him to anyone she knew. She said he was not just a good doctor he was a good person. I thanked her for sharing her story with me. She may be the reason I want to share my story because she really inspired me. Meeting Mary reminds me of a Wisdom Quote I recently read, "In life, you will realize there is a role for everyone you meet. Some will test you, some will use you, some will love you, and some will teach you. But the ones who are truly important are the ones who bring out the best in you. They are the rare and amazing people who remind you why it's worth it."

I also found a wonderful masseuse while getting a massage with my daughter Jessie. When I told her I recently had mastectomy surgery she proceeded to give me the gentlest and most caring massage I have ever had. The massage included a warm towel for my feet and special oil for my nose to help my sinuses. One of the most unexpected places where I found a kind person was at the dermatologist office. She gave me a discount on the broken veins on my breasts and skin tag removal after I told her I had the broken veins because my skin was stretched to put in a breast implant. She and her assistant could not have been nicer and when I went to pay the bill I was charged for only one skin tag removal instead of three. It is good to know there will be always be many more people who are kind in this world than people who are unkind.

I read about a wonderfully kind woman who I will probably never meet. She is a tattoo artist who puts tattoos on breasts which are scarred after breast cancer surgery, she does nipple tattoos free of charge. I really am glad there are people in the world like this tattoo artist who care enough about women with breast cancer to think of a way to make them feel beautiful. I am not sure if I will ever be brave enough to get such a tattoo. If I do I hope it is someone kind and caring like the tattoo artist I read about. They showed pictures of some of her work and she had tattooed beautiful flowers, pink ribbons and various other designs over her client's breast cancer scars. I am sure the women she has tattooed are very grateful for the wonderful things she has done for their scarred and battered bodies. When I read her story I was reminded of this quote: "Cancer tried to knock me down but my determination to fight to win is non-negotiable. I want to see the sunrise, the sunset and experience all the seasons that life has to offer. I want a lifetime of it. It's doing what I need to do to experience the next sunrise, the next sunset and the next season."

~Ann—LymphomaClub.Com

It May Be Contagious

*T*HANK GOODNESS I have had many people who have shown me kindness and love during my breast cancer journey. But I also want to discuss people who were not so kind. The people who have treated me badly will have to be forgiven because holding a grudge is a form of hate and it only hurts the person who holds onto it. As Maya Angelou has said, "Hate causes a lot of problems in this world, but has not solved one yet." So I have decided instead of holding a grudge against someone it is easier for me to cut them out of my life. I will decide if the time we spend together is worth the hurt or disappointment they inflict on me. I will not expect anything from the people who disappointed me because I know I will be disappointed again by them. So instead of worrying about the next time they will hurt me I will move ahead without them in my life. There are too many wonderful people in the world to waste your time being around people who are negative and hurtful. I found a great quote about being disappointed and hurt by friends and/or relatives from Wisdom Quotes: "No one can promise they'll never hurt you because one time or another they will. The real promise is the time you spend together will be worth the pain." So the people who have disappointed me will be judged on the time we spend together. Is that time worth the pain they inflict on me? Or do I need to cut them out of my life and move on?

The first person who was a big disappointment to me was a relative who proclaimed how much she loved me, and how concerned about me she was yet she did not come to visit once or did not even bother to call me. She texted me twice saying she was coming to visit. The first time she made up a weird excuse and the second time she just did not show up and gave no explanation. She did leave a message three weeks afterwards and invited me to dinner. I just ignored her message. I did not want to go down that road again. I was afraid she would make plans for dinner and then text me at the last minute and cancel the plans. She reminds me of a quote I saw on Facebook the other day. The quote said, "When someone treats you like and option, help them narrow their choices by removing yourself from the equation, it is that simple," Wisdom Quotes. I just want to say to her and people like her: do not promise someone that you will come and visit them when you really do not have any intentions of doing so. If you do it to make yourself feel better it is a very selfish thing for you to do. Instead stop and think how bad you are making the person on the receiving end of your "promise" feel. If you do not want to see someone who looks ill or if you are afraid they will talk about themselves and their illness too much and you will be repulsed or bored out of your mind, then just wait until a few weeks after surgery and invite them to dinner or a movie. Most people would much prefer something like dinner or a movie to a false promise. I know it was an extremely hurtful experience for me when my relative promised they would visit but they did not. The fact is I did not need false promises because I had people who came to visit me after my surgeries. I also had people who could not come to visit me but instead called or sent cards. I think the person making false promises tells themselves, "Well I tried to come over and she just did not understand I was too tired or _____ (insert your excuse here) to show up." As Wisdom Quotes says, "If it is important to you, you will find a way. If not you will find an excuse."

Another disappointing person was a friend I had known since elementary school. When I called to tell her about my first surgery she cried so hard she had to hang up and call me back, which really touched me. As time progressed that one display of sympathy could not outweigh everything else she did. In other words her actions spoke much louder than her words. She came to visit me once when she was up for the holidays. It was after my first surgery and she gave me a Christmas present however she said she could "only stay a minute." She had an accident a couple months after I had my first surgery. She was confined to bed. She would call and say, "You never want to go through something like this it is awful." I would think, "Really you think your problem is worse than cancer?" She did have to stay in bed for months so I knew she was in a lot of pain. I normally would have sent her flowers or candy however since she did not send me anything after I had my surgery (before her accident). I decided not to send a single thing to her either. I know it may sound childish however I really did not feel like making an effort with her anymore. I dreaded talking to her and began ignoring her calls and very rarely returned any of her calls. I could not stand to listen to her and her pity party full of excuses. Instead of calling her I wrote letters updating her on my condition. After my second mastectomy she sent a get well card and on it she wrote, "Call me anytime we have been so busy here, lots going on." To me this message screamed, "I am just kidding do not call me I am too busy to talk to you." So the excuses began. She waited two months to call me and when she did call (I was screening her calls so she had to leave a message) she left a message saying, "This second surgery of yours has been so hard on me and I do not know what to say to you because I am not taking it well." She was not taking it well? How did she think I was taking it? I really did not feel like comforting her. I guess she wanted to call me to tell me about all the pain my surgeries had caused her. I needed comforting! I was not about to call and comfort her. I felt like she was just making excuses so she would not have to deal with me. When someone starts making excuses

I have learned they make them for themselves so they can feel better about themselves. She said she could not visit me because she does not drive and is dependent on someone to bring her to my house which is two hours away. Somehow she managed to make it to a local mall near my house and when she saw me at the mall she was embarrassed. She stammered, "I did not call you to tell you I was in town because I am only going to be here for a day," and there is it is another excuse to be a bad friend. After seeing her at the mall I thought, "Wow she is a terrible friend." When I had my second breast removed I wrote her a letter telling her what was going on with me. I knew she was coming to this area because she said during an earlier conversation that she and her husband were coming up for a wedding. She neither came to visit nor called when she was just a few miles from my house. I really cannot imagine not going to visit her if our places where switched and she had breast cancer instead of me. I think that hurts most of all. Because she did not do anything special for me I stopped wanting to do anything for her. I could have gone to visit her when she was in bed for a couple months with her injury. Because she showed no interest in coming to see I really felt no desire to visit her. I now feel she is not really a friend as a matter of fact most of the time she seems more like a stranger. I will continue to send birthday and Christmas gifts to her because she sends them to me and will continue to write back to her when she sends a card. Unfortunately our friendship did not stand the test of time. I need to have people in my life who really care about me. I recently found a quote which describes exactly the way I think she feels about me. The quote says, "Grieving is suddenly contagious if you come to close you might catch my bad luck," from Sing you Home by Jodi Picoult. I believe she thought I had bad luck and she did not want to be around me because of it. I also think she knew I would be grieving over the loss of my breasts and she could not deal with my grief. My illness was a true test of my friendships and only the strong friends have survived the test.

My Family and Friends

I DID HAVE many strong friends and family who survived the test of my illness. They did wonderful things for me and made me feel better about myself too. Oprah Winfrey said, "Surround yourself with people who lift you up because there are too many people in this world who want to bring you down." So many people have done wonderful things for me during my cancer journey. My oldest daughter, my youngest daughter, my hubby and my son-in-law, David came to my first surgery and took care of me when I came home. They even tried to help me when I passed out from the pain. I remember being up in my bedroom with pain coming in waves over my entire body. But when I heard the sound of my two daughters in the kitchen laughing while they prepared dinner I was blissfully happy. I felt like I had a happy home and I was a lucky mama. The laughter between them lifted my spirits and made me happier than they will ever know.

After my second mastectomy my daughter Jessie and our grandson, Caleb came over and spent the night. The joy they brought to me and continue to bring to me is "priceless." To watch a baby grow under the loving care of his mother is something which brings me such happiness. I was very thankful my daughter Jessie brought my grandson over to visit with me during the hard times, after the surgeries and during the recoveries. He makes me laugh and forget about all my problems for a moment or two he is good for my soul. My daughter Jessie also requested prayer for me and she asked her in-laws to pray for me on my surgery days. It always makes me feel good when someone who has a good connection with the man upstairs puts a good word in for me.

My friend Dessie also prayed for me a lot. I had not met her when I had my first surgery I told her about all my surgeries after we got to know each other. She requested prayer for me at her church and she prayed for me also. She was great to have around after my second surgery because when we got together for lunch we did not talk about cancer; we were too busy catching up on our lives. She invited me to her church and we frequently met for lunch which gave me something to look forward to. She also invited me to see the Hunger Games movie with her female friends from church and we had so much fun making a Hunger Games themed lunch before the movie. Everyone brought a Hunger Games themed dish to share. We ate our yummy lunch in a beautifully restored Victorian mansion owned by Dessie's friend. Then we went to see the movie. Fun was had by all.

My friend Jennifer has been great also she continues to send sweet and caring emails and she came over right after my first surgery with yummy food. She even sat and looked at me without shock on her face when she saw how gray and scary I looked. During my last surgery she was in Ireland so she could not bring me a yummy dinner. Instead she bought an Irish teapot for me while she was in Ireland. She surprised me with it when we both attended a luncheon. It was such a touching and caring thing for her to do! I still have that Irish teapot on display in my china cabinet.

Other visitors I had were friends Harold and Jean. They came over after both of my surgeries and brought homemade dinners and desserts and shared them with my husband and myself. Because Harold had cancer ten years prior to mine they can both relate to what I was going through. It was so nice to have a normal dinner at home with such good friends. It made me feel like one day my life would get back to normal. Jean has also sent me tons of encouraging emails and she sat with me and ate Bourbon cheesecake before my second mastectomy. Doing normal things like eating cheesecake and chatting meant so much to me.

Some people did not come to see me immediately after my surgery. When they did it ended up being just the right time. My friend Roberta did not come to see me immediately after my first surgery. She did email me during my recovery. A few months later she came to my house for a visit. When she came she brought a dozen of her old tea pots. She knows I love all things tea related and that I collect old and new teapots. I was touched by her thoughtfulness.

My niece Angie who lives in Texas called and asked me if I would rather she came up to see me before or after my first surgery. At the time I thought she should come before my surgery. I did not tell her because I could tell she wanted to come up after my surgery when I felt better. I now realize it was so much better for her to come afterwards because we were able to attend events I would not have been able to attend immediately after my first surgery. We went to an historical tea with my daughter Jessie. We got to eat in a beautiful Victorian style home and after lunch we took a bus to explore more historical homes. We also went to a Christmas dinner at our local Historical Society. We had such fun and she got to see snow for the first time in a long time (since she lives in Houston, TX). She was so excited to walk in the snow. It was so good for me to get out and do things I love to do with my niece. When I took her to the airport to return home she cried so hard and said she loved me. It touched my heart.

I was also pleasantly surprised my three brothers (they are the brothers from my adopted family) called me frequently during my recovery. We were never close because there was such a big difference in our ages. I was just a kid about eight years old when they all left home and after they left home they did not come around much. The two oldest brothers live in other states and the youngest brother lives two hours away and works a lot of overtime hours however he has been great about calling and checking on me.

My youngest sister came to visit after my first surgery brought flowers and a card and called to check on me after both surgeries. We had not had much contact for years but because of my breast cancer she got back in contact with me. She is my blood sister; she was also the child of Kaye and Bob (our birth parents) and like me she was adopted by my aunt and her family. She was adopted by them a year after I was adopted. They adopted her when she was nine months old. She was not a healthy child and was in an orphanage. My adopted parents did not wait till she was two years old to adopt her like they had waited to adopt me. They said they were afraid if they did not adopt her when they did she would not have lived much longer. She was very sick and had severe diarrhea. When she and I were adopted the house was full. We had three brothers and an older sister: six kids and two adults. Later it seemed like my youngest sister and I were the only kids in the family because our four adopted siblings had already left home by the time I was eight. The older kids moved out and were busy with their lives. My older sister attended many Holiday parties at our house with her husband and four kids before she moved to Texas. My brothers did not come around as much. Even though my adopted sister is eight years older than me our lives were very similar. She left home when I was eight so she could get married at the age of 16; I married young too at the age of 18. My adopted sister raised four kids and was married for over 40 years, before she got a divorce; I raised two kids and have been married over 38 years. She and I both raised our kids in the "traditional" American family way. Back in our day it was the norm to raise our kids with the same man and stay married to that man all of your life. Our lives were similar so I felt we had a lot more in common than my younger sister and I did.

I felt my adopted mother favored my youngest sister and did not really care for me. My youngest sister and I always seem to have an unspoken rivalry over who our adopted mother liked the most and in my mind my youngest sister always won. Once she got a divorce I could not relate to her because she dated and was a single parent. I watched her youngest son anytime she needed me to so she could go out on dates. He was a sweet boy and got along great with my daughter Jessie. After they both moved thousands of miles away I lost contact with them. I sent letters and tried to call them however they moved a lot and changed their phone number frequently. Even when she moved back to a city near me we did not try to keep in touch. We just did not seem to have anything in common. When she heard about my cancer she immediately called and asked if she could come over. After that first visit she called and checked on me but as time went on we again drifted apart.

My Brother Timmy

ETWEEN MY FIRST and second mastectomy my brother Timmy found out he had cancer. I called him on occasion to check on him. I sent him cards and I made plans to visit him when he felt well enough to receive visitors. He had to have chemotherapy and it was a hard road for him. He had stage-four lymphoma and was very weak and lost a lot of weight. I do not think I was as good about calling him as he was about calling me. I am more of a letter and card person. I was glad to hear he had lots of friends and family who were concerned about him and his wife took good care of him. Once when he called me to check on my breast cancer status he started telling me about his cancer journey and I realized I was not the only one who had trouble with their doctors. He went to his local VA hospital (he was a veteran of the Vietnam War) because he was losing weight and had a sore throat and swollen glands. They told him he had allergies and gave him medicine and sent him on his way. He kept losing weight and feeling sick so he decided to get a second opinion. The doctor told him she needed to run tests and when she got those test results back she told him the results showed he had Hodgkin's lymphoma. He was shocked and dismayed because he had been on allergy medicine for a year which was prescribed by the VA hospital. He had always assumed his nausea was due to the side effects of the Agent Orange which was sprayed in the jungles while he was a soldier fighting in Vietnam. By the time he was diagnosed correctly his cancer was in stage four so the doctor told him he immediately had to get chemotherapy and possibly radiation. When he got the bill from the second doctor he knew he could not afford go to another doctor who was not covered under the VA medical plan. He gathered all of his medical records including the first diagnosis at the original VA hospital and the second opinion results. He then traveled to a VA hospital in another state which all his friends had told him was the best one around. It was four hours from where he lived. He traveled those four hours to get free medical care from the VA hospital because he knew he could not afford to pay doctor bills. He did not have any other kind of health insurance. When he got to the hospital he had to fight to be treated for his cancer. He went there and told them he was not leaving until someone saw him. He waited for about an hour until the hospital found a room and gave him fluids through an IV. They kept him in the hospital for a week. They told him if he had not arrived at the hospital when he did he would have died that day. He was severely dehydrated because he could not keep anything in his stomach. He had also lost a lot of weight and was very weak. After he was in the hospital for a week they sent him home with anti-nausea medicine and told him he needed to put on some weight and get stronger. Once he did that they would begin chemotherapy. He ate as much as he could and built his strength back up to start chemotherapy. They had to stop giving him chemotherapy a couple times because he grew too weak. Once he got built back up they started all over again. He had radiation treatments and hoped between that and the chemotherapy the cancer would be gone and he would go into remission. My sisters and I went in October 2012, to visit him at Hope House in Nashville, TN. We had a wonderful visit and I am so happy we got to go. The sad fact is if the VA doctors would have diagnosed him correctly years ago he would not have been in stage four when they found his cancer. His original diagnosis was inaccurate and the medicines they gave him at the previous VA hospital were not doing the job of healing him or making him feel better. I am sad to report he died of Lymphoma cancer in December 2012. We had his funeral on New Year's Eve and we mourn his passing every day. He was a perfect example of someone who aggressively sought out accurate medical attention.

Cancer and My Future Health

I HAVE HAD so many surgeries which included many doses of anesthesia. The doctor explained to me sometimes the anesthesia and antibiotics kills the good bacteria in my stomach and that is why I have a lot of issues with my stomach. A lot of the good bacteria in my stomach are gone and now it is rebelling. We fixed the cancer issues now I have new issues. Every time I see a new doctor for a checkup or if I have an injury they always want to know about my cancer. They want to know if I had radiation or chemotherapy. They take my cancer into consideration no matter why I come to see them. I recently hurt my back while on a boat. After we hit a wake hard I could not stand up and had trouble breathing. When I went to see a specialist she looked at the paperwork I filled out and the first thing she asked was not, "how does your back feel," instead she wanted to know all about my breast cancer. She explained some breast cancer treatments make bones in the body weak and she was wondering if that was what caused the compression fracture in my back. I did not have radiation or chemotherapy so it was not an issue with me. I know for many women weakening bones is a side effect of their cancer treatments. She was also concerned my cancer had come back and moved to my bones, which is another common problem for women with any kind of cancer. My cancer will always effect what kind of treatment doctors suggest for an injury or illness. Cancer is not something I can just forget about. I know when I have a broken bone or a fracture the doctors will check to see if the cancer has returned and gotten to my bones to make them weak and brittle. In this case it was not cancer. It is frightening because I will always have to wonder "if." In the back of my mind "if" will always be there. Thank goodness I have people who will be by my side to support me.

It is so good to have friends and family who show me by their words and deeds how much they love me. Some people I love and some who I thought were my friends disappointed and hurt me. I saw an anonymous quote on Facebook which said, "Do not blame people for disappointing you blame yourself for expecting too much from them." I do not think I agree with that quote. I think we expect people we love to behave as if they love us or at least care about us when we go through good or bad times. I have had both wonderful experiences and not so wonderful experiences with friends, family and doctors throughout my ordeal. I feel all of these experiences have helped me through this cancer journey. I have learned to accept my cancer. I have also learned telling the world I am a survivor is good for me.

I have discovered it is okay to let people know I am a breast cancer survivor. After my first surgery I wanted to keep my cancer to myself, no pink shirts and "Save the Boobies" banners for me. I did not want people to ask me questions so I did not wear pink or talk about breast cancer. I did not want to stand out as the "sad person who had cancer." However I did attend a Breast Cancer walk in Dayton, OH in 2011 with daughter Jessie and we walked and ate pink ribbon cookies and had a great time. The next year I could not attend the walk because I was out of town but my daughter Jessie walked with my grandson and her husband. It made me very happy they would care enough about me to do the cancer walk. After going through mastectomy surgery a second time I realized people do not always make a fuss when you have surgery. Actually sometimes it is just the opposite, some just do not care. One relative asked me why I was so secretive about my first surgery, she complained, "I found out a year later." So to make amends I told her ahead of time that I was getting a second mastectomy surgery. What was her reaction, nothing no card, no call, no visits. I felt like I should have done what I did the first time and not tell her anything for a year or so. When I first got breast cancer I knew some people would not care and it hurts more and is much more disappointing to have people not care than to have people ask questions and show concern! I have decided I do not want to protect myself from other people's lack of concern. I do not want to hide my cancer just in case people do not care. I am more eager to share my cancer battle with people. I drive around with a "Cure Breast Cancer" license plate and I wear a lot of pink and carry a pink purse. When people tell me they love my purse, which they often do, I proudly tell them I bought it on-line at the Breast Cancer web site. I post comments on Facebook and I read about breast cancer research and am eager to learn more about what causes the disease and how we can find a cure. I love this quote about cancer, "We won't just survive we will thrive," the Breast Cancer Website.

In 2012 I attended a lecture on breast health with my friend Jean. It was a presentation by a local oncologist and it was funded by a local hospital. The hospital provided dinner and the setting was the local country club. I found some very enlightening information about my cancer at his presentation. He talked about the various stages of cancer and he said Stage zero breast cancer is not even considered cancer. He said it is considered a breast disease. He said for someone with Stage zero he would recommend a lumpectomy not a mastectomy. He said the downside of a lumpectomy would be the possibility of needing radiation therapy or chemotherapy afterwards. Also there would be a possibility the patient would have to be tested every six to twelve months for reoccurring cancer. He said most likely the tests would include a biopsy, an MRI or a mammogram. There was also a possibility the patient might have to have all three. I was startled by the information he gave us at the lecture. I really feel like the two oncologists I saw should have told me everything the oncologist at the presentation did.

Everything he said made sense because when I first found out about my breast cancer (yes I am going to continue to call it cancer) my surgeon cheerfully announced he had "good news." He said I did not have breast cancer instead I had what he called "pre-cancer." The oncologist doing the presentation I attended had gone even further than my surgeon. This oncologist called what I had "breast disease." He did not call it cancer. As a matter of fact he said breast disease was not cancer. But no matter what the doctors call it, I still had to have a mastectomy and that is a pretty serious consequence of a "breast disease." I guess if I would have gone to this particular oncologist before my first mastectomy he would have suggest I have a lumpectomy and not a mastectomy. But who knows how that would have turned out.

I also got confirmation at the presentation that because my cancer was just considered a breast disease and not breast cancer and because I was older than 50 when I acquired this "disease" my daughters did not have to be overly concerned about getting breast cancer due to heredity. He did say the daughters of women with breast cancer or breast disease would need to subtract 10 years from whatever age their mother first found their breast cancer or disease. This number would be the year the daughters would need to have their first breast exam. So since I found my breast cancer at 54 my daughters would need to have their first breast exam at age 44. Continuing to learn more about breast cancer not only helps me understand what happened to me. It also helps me keep my daughters informed about what they need to do to make sure they do not get breast cancer. They need to have early checkups and keep informed on their breast health. My daughters are amazing ladies and I want their lives to be happy and healthy. My youngest is such a good mother to her son and she volunteers by scuba diving in the Manatee tanks at the zoo and my oldest is a writer and published her first book, <u>Couple Friends</u>, last year. They both have busy fulfilling lives and I do not want their lives to be overshadowed by cancer. They do have to be more careful just because I had "breast disease." In the meantime I do not want any of us to dwell on the negative side of breast cancer I want us to find the joys in life and hold onto them tightly.

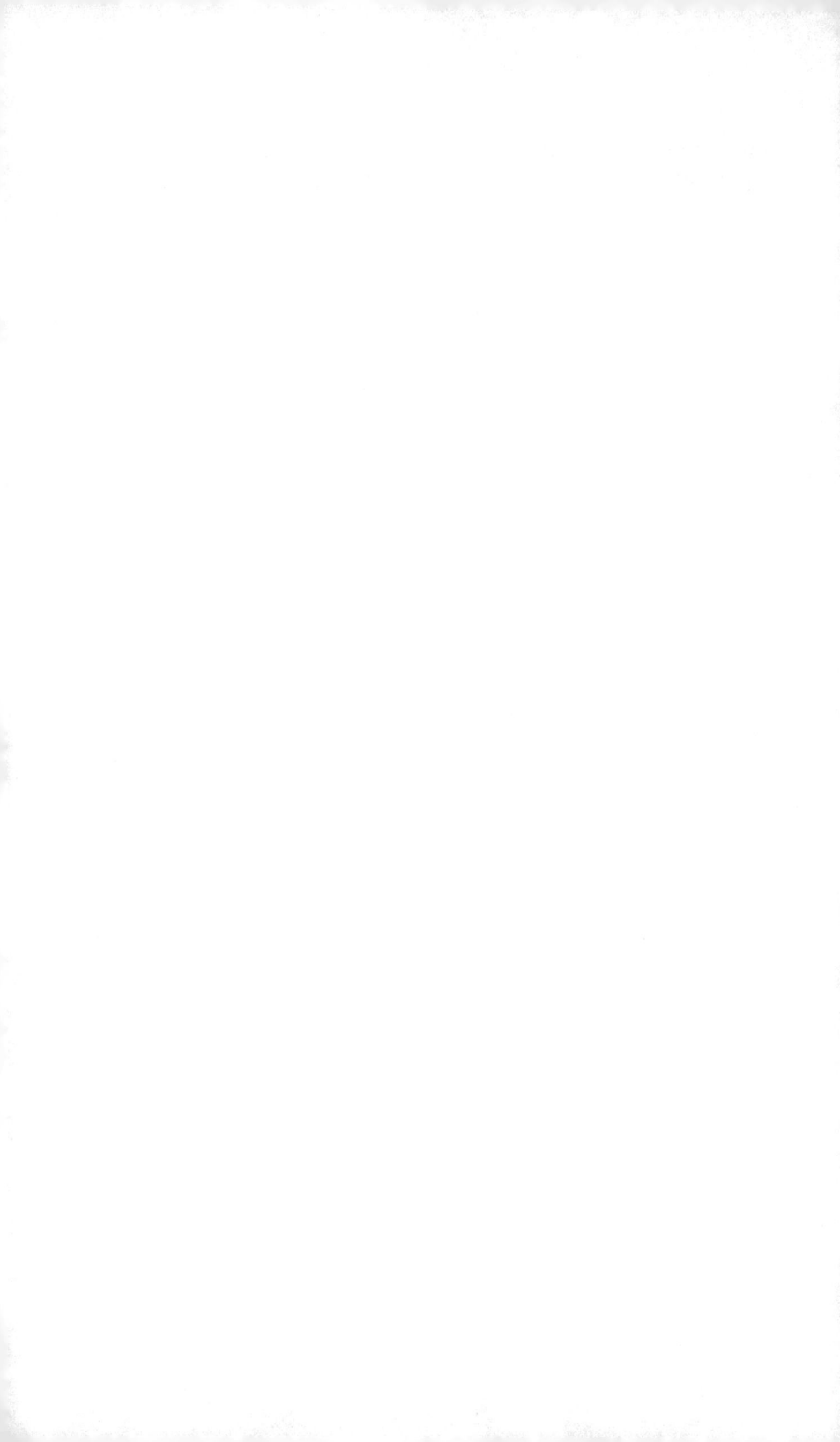

Our Vacation Home

ONE JOY IN my life is our vacation home in Florida. When we first bought the fixer upper house five years ago the two of us did not seem to treat the Florida house like a vacation home. In the beginning we were so busy fixing the house up inside and out we did not feel like we were on vacation when we were there. There were walls to paint, furniture to buy, tile floors to be installed, wood floors to be installed, and curtains to buy and hang. The landscaping in Florida grew like crazy because of the warm weather. So we always had work to do around the house. It seemed like every time we went to our house for a "vacation" we were spending money and working on the house most of the time.

When we go on a cruise or stay at a hotel we do not have to clean or spend money fixing something. We get to enjoy our entire vacation relaxing. In Florida we were always working. Once we got the majority of the updating done we thought we could go down to our house and actually take a vacation. Because we were at our house we did not have the luxury of maids and room service so we had to go to the grocery, do laundry, cook a lot of meals ourselves etc. We also did not treat our time in Florida like it was a vacation. We did not plan things to do like a normal vacation. We got into a rut of waking up eating, watching TV and making a "need to buy/

do list." The only vacation thing we did was walk on the beach every day and a lot of times we only walked on the beach so we would get out of the house for some exercise. My husband works a lot and we are not used to having so much time together without a vacation itinerary. He normally works 72 hours a week. So to go from never seeing each other when we are home to being together 24/7 when we are in Florida was quite an adjustment for us. Finally I realized we were stressed out because we were not used to being together so much. When I shared this observation with my husband he agreed this was the problem. We began working on being more patient with each other. I do not complain that he sleeps in everyday and he takes me out to eat a lot. We make a list of "fun things to do" and we plan our days so we have something to look forward to every day. We try to make our visits to Florida more like a normal vacation and less like our regular everyday life. We still walk on the beach for an hour every evening. We enjoy the walks so much more than when we first bought the Florida house. Now when we are there we find peace and we just feel so at home. As Kenny Chesney says, "We all need to find a place where we find peace."

When I hear the ocean I immediately relax. It is such a soothing sound and we are lucky to have found a small but cozy place where we can go to for a nice vacation once or twice a year until we retire there. Our vacation home is only half the size of the home we live in now. It has a sunroom which makes the house seem much bigger than it really is. The yard is small compared to the 28 acres where we currently live. Our lot in Florida is on a corner so it is a bigger lot than most on our street. It is located in a subdivision. At the Florida cottage we are at the end of the street at an intersection. The two streets which surround our house have very little traffic; usually just the neighbor's cars go by. The house was built in the 50's so it has survived a lot of hurricanes, tropical storms and just plain crazy Florida weather. I really love the six palm trees and the beautiful flowering privacy hedge, a cactus, robin nest ferns and many other tropical plants. All of this wonderful foliage was already here so I did not have to plant it! When we look out the front window we see the beautiful centerpiece that the former owners planted for privacy. It includes a palm tree and tall tropical foliage. We see lovely greenery instead of cars going down the street or the neighbor's houses. So even though we do not have 28 acres to hide behind at our Florida home we still have a sense of seclusion even with the front drapes open. There is also bright pink bougainvillea and white jasmine growing up the lattice on the Florida back porch, which gives a sense of privacy when we sit there to enjoy the weather. Back porches are a wonderful place to sit and contemplate life. When I sit on the Florida porch in May the smell of jasmine in bloom is heaven sent. So even though our cottage is half the size of our regular home, it is going to be perfect for us when we retire. I am looking forward to having less space to clean and hoard things. There is so much stuff in our full time house which really needs to be thrown away. For some reason I hoard it thinking, "Someday I may need this." With the girls married and gone we do not need so much space. Our little cottage is a slice of heaven. Our Florida cottage reminds me of a quote, "I need sometime in a beautiful place to help me clear my head," Wisdom Quotes. Our cottage in Florida is definitely such a place.

One of the joys I find in life is traveling. I look forward to each trip I take and after every trip I start planning my next trip. I also run a sports team travel business so I plan those trips and usually go on the trips as a guide. I find it exciting to travel. Planning and anticipating my trips are half the fun of traveling. We have always loved to travel as a family. We used to go to Daytona Beach almost every year when the kids were growing up. We would get a hotel room which had a mini kitchen and we would save money by eating breakfast and lunch in our room. We took a cruise with both daughters and our son in law, Gary to the Caribbean in 2003. In 2007 we cruised with our daughter Shawndra and her husband to Alaska. We have also been on a family vacation to Cancun, Mexico. We always loved our family vacations and really looked forward to them every year. When we first became empty nesters

I thought the two of us would never enjoy traveling without our daughters. Our daughters have always been so much fun to travel with and I was afraid we would be lonely without them as travel companions. We have learned to love traveling alone and since we both love to travel we find cruises are the easiest way to go. We love it because activities are planned; food and entertainment are provided so we do not have to do a lot of work. We actually get to relax. Any kind of travel is good for me, as Rumi said, "Travel brings power and love back you're your life."

We traveled to our Florida home in July 2012 and went to see the local fireworks they show every year on the river near our vacation home. The beauty of the fireworks over the river cannot be described with words. A person has to see these fireworks for themselves. This makes the third year we have traveled to Florida just to see the fireworks. We also got to see our daughter Shawndra and her husband while we were in Florida it is always a joy to see them. We have a favorite restaurant there which makes the best bruschetta. They also have Martini night specials every Wednesday night so we always make a trip to that restaurant when we go down to our cottage in Florida. We also walk by the ocean every night when we are in Florida and when I am by the ocean I truly feel all the worries of life are washed away with the sound of each crashing wave. The ocean really renews me. I feel blessed we found a small cottage by the ocean we can visit whenever we need to feel renewed.

We took another trip to Florida in September of 2012. We vacationed with our daughter Jessie, our grandson Caleb and Jessie's husband David. Mark and I flew down while Jessie and her family drove down. We went to the beach, out to eat and also to Marine Land near St. Augustine. It was a joy to see Caleb's face the first time he saw the ocean. He loved everything about the ocean. He also loved using his walker to fly all over our tile floors. He was a happy vacation baby. We also went to Savannah and visited with Shawndra and Gary. We took them out to eat and hung out all day with them. It was so nice to be together as a family. Being able to be with Caleb on his first visit to the ocean was priceless. Jessie and I wanted to go see the dolphin from the movie "A Dolphin Tail" however we ran out of time and did not get to travel to St Petersburg to see it. We saw the movie in the spring and found out the dolphin was in an aquarium which was not far from our Florida house. The movie is about a dolphin who gets hit by a boat and his tail gets cut off in the accident. The scientists who rescued him make an artificial tail for him so he can swim. It was an uplifting movie of survival. The story really warmed my heart since I am also a survivor. Even though we did not get to see the dolphin we had a blast in Florida and it a precious memory I will never forget. Going to Florida also means wearing a swimsuit if I go to the ocean. I used to dread the thought of going in the ocean however my breasts match better now. I have two silicone implants which almost match. It is not such a challenge to find swimsuits and blouses which fit. I feel lucky to be alive and lucky to have a life blessed with friends, family and travel. I think people should find what gives them joy in life and go for it. As long as your joy does not cause pain or harm to yourself or to others.

The Good Things in Life

*S*OMETHING ELSE WHICH brings me joy is sitting on my back porch at our full time house and listening to the wind blowing in the trees and the birds chirping. I sit out and read and drink tea or I bring out my laptop and have a cocktail. Sometimes I work on my business website while sitting outside on the porch. It is especially nice in the spring and fall when it is not too hot. My husband moved a freestanding swing to our porch and now when our grandson comes to visit, I hold him in my lap and sing to him while we swing. He is fascinated by the chains on the swing. He gets so excited watching them sway back and forth. After a while though he gets sleepy and usually falls asleep while I hold him. Between the swaying of the chains and my singing his little eyes cannot stay open and he is asleep in my arms. It gives me peace to look into the beautiful face of my baby grandson Caleb. He is such a pleasure and joy to have around and I am so excited to watch him grow and become a good person. He has a great mommy (my daughter, Jessie) and a wonderful father so he is one lucky little man. When I rocked him to sleep the other day before his nap I looked down at him curled up in my arms and sucking his thumb and I thought how thankful I am to God for letting me have another baby in my life to love and be a Nana to. I feel so happy when he is around. I have so much fun watching him try to talk, eat, crawl and laugh. Just doing little things with him is so much fun. We took Caleb out to dinner the other night. I loved watching the joy on his face when he tried new foods, watched other customers, and got attention from a waiter. He loved to look up at the beautiful lights above our table. He can make a simple trip to a restaurant an adventure. The joy of a grandchild is an amazing experience for me.

I am lucky to have a grandson to enjoy and play with. I am also lucky that I get to travel to so many exciting places. Visiting with my grandson and the thought of future travel keeps my mind off of my problems and gives me something to look forward to. There are quite a few things other things I have found which help me keep my mind off my cancer and the IBS resulting from all my surgeries. One of them is watching Sex and The City reruns. I love Carrie and I love days when they have a marathon of the Sex and the City. Even though I would never want to be any of the four girls on the show, I do want to have a real life version of their fictional friendships. I love how they stick by each other's side. Sometimes they fight and do not talk to each other for days on end. Sometimes they get on each other's last nerve and need a break however they always remain true friends. I have always wanted to have friendships like the ones the women in Sex in the City enjoy.

Friendships are very important but when you are sick having a wonderful doctor is very important. My GYN is a wonderful doctor who showed such concern and caring both times I went through my ordeal. He has been my doctor for over 20 years and he never ceases to be a great and caring man. The people who did the breast biopsy and my MD were wonderful. They never gave up trying to help me until I got the tests completed. I thank them for their professionalism and concern. I am also glad I had a wonderful plastic surgeon. My surgeon, Dr. Han, had skilled hands and a wonderful bedside manner. He listened to me when I had questions. He was patient, calm and cool and had answers to such questions as, "Why do people insisted on telling me I should not have surgery" or "Why do people think they know more than my own doctors?" He is a great doctor and he performed miracles with my implants and my multiple surgeries.

I also have prayed a lot during this time and I feel I have grown closer to God. I have asked God this question a time or two, "Why me Lord, what awful things have I done to deserve this?" I have to allow myself to question everything that has happened and even to question God because without questioning life a person does not learn lessons from it. I have learned many lessons and I hope to use them to make my life and other people's lives better. It has been wonderful to pray a silent prayer and cry tears of thankfulness because God has given me more years to live. As Mae West said, "You only live once, but if you do it right, once is enough." Another favorite quote which I love and which I feel applies to my breast cancer journey (even though the author was not speaking on breast cancer):

> "If there is anything to take away from this . . . it's the reminder that life is very fragile. Our time here is limited and it is precious. And what matters at the end of the day is not the small things, it's not the trivial things, which so often consume us and our daily lives. Ultimately, it is how we choose to treat one another and how we love one another."—President Barack Obama

I am sure over the years I have not always treated someone who was ill or sick in the way they would have liked to have been treated. I usually send flowers and cards however I am not the best at being by someone's side. So I probably have not done everything I should have for one person or another. I want to say I am sorry if I was not the friend you needed me to be. I am thankful I have been given another chance to treat people in my life better.

Thank You

I HOPE WRITING this book not only helps make my life better I also hope it helps others with their breast cancer journey. Writing this book made me realize the reason I did not want to tell people about my cancer was because I was protecting myself from the hurt inflicted by people who would show no concern for me. People who would basically not care one way or another about the pain I was going through. Admitting that is something that I really did not want to include in my book. When I decided to write this book, I wanted to include everything I went through during my cancer journey: the good, the bad and the ugly. I hope reading this book will make people stop and think before they say something negative to a person who has had cancer or any kind of illness. People with chronic illnesses have been through enough so be kind. Think about the pain this person is going through and do not add to their suffering!

I am thankful for people who have lifted me up during my cancer journey and who are not afraid to tell their stories to the world and for people like my nurse Mary who shared her story of survival. I think we all need to read encouraging stories about someone who has gone through something terrible like breast cancer, someone who came out the other side with a wonderful story and a wonderful attitude. I love reading about Movie stars and Television stars who have survived their cancer battles. It makes me stronger. I also love to read books about regular people like me who have battled cancer. Our stories of survival let people know cancer can be beaten. We may feel like we have been beaten up physically and mentally after our cancer battles however we have to remember this:

What cancer cannot do
It cannot make us less of a woman
It cannot make us a bad person
It cannot make our children love us less
It cannot change the wonderful memories we have

What cancer can do
It can make us stronger if we let it
It can make us cry
It can change our lives forever
It is up to us to decide, do we let it change our lives for better or for worse?

I am also writing this book to try and let women know they are not alone. I want to let them know they need to fight to get quality care from doctors. Do not let the doctors tell you something you know does not sound right. Do research and get a second, third or fourth opinion. Let the world know you had cancer and survived. Cancer is not a punishment distributed by God. It is just cancer and something which a person has to work through. I know working through cancer made me a stronger person.

Another lesson I learned during my cancer journey which I would like to share is: do not go to a breast cancer specialty store to buy your bras and breast form inserts. I spent $1700.00 on a specialty bra and silicone breast forms. I ended up rarely wearing them because they were too heavy and made my back hurt due to the extra weight. The woman at the shop convinced me I needed three forms to make my breasts match. I know a lot of women who have no insurance or who are like me and only receive partial insurance coverage for the cost of reconstruction brassieres and accessories. I could not return anything I purchased because the policy posted on the dressing room door is, "Once you take it home it cannot be returned." So even though I could not wear the expensive silicone breast forms I did wear the $100.00 bra. I ended up spending $1700.00 and could only wear the $100.00 bra. Take my advice and try TLC on line before you go to a specialty store. I ended up buying nice foam inserts from TLC online at about $25 per form. Instead of three breast forms I need two, one to wear and one to use as a backup. I washed one and wore one. Besides the great price of the breast forms on TLC I was happy to learn I could wash them on a regular basis and they came out smelling great versus the silicone forms that I had to hand wash. No matter how many times I washed the silicone forms they never felt clean. We live and learn and when we share the things we learn we can help other people to avoid the mistakes we made.

I am excited to share information about a program I recently participated in called BRA. It is a reconstruction campaign to support breast cancer survivor's right to be informed and choose whether breast reconstruction following mastectomy is right for them. The pop singer Jewel is the spokeswoman for this campaign. The article on-line at GLOBE NEWSWIRE said, "Today, the American Society of Plastic Surgeons and The Plastic Surgery Foundation announced their partnership with New York Breast Reconstruction Alliance (nyBRA) in support of the first national Breast Reconstruction Awareness (BRA) Day USA, October 17, 2012. Their goal is to help women who are not informed of their reconstructive options after mastectomies. Research shows seven out of 10 women diagnosed with breast cancer are not informed of their options. The U.S. and 20 other countries joined together for BRA Day on October 17, 2012. On that day my daughter Shawndra and I participated in BRA Day in Daytona Beach, FL. At the walk many women decorated their bras and wore them outside of their shirts. They had a turn-out of about 10,000 people it was an amazing wall of pink. Someone even put their pit bull in a pink tutu. At the end of the walk there was a choir of young men singing wonderful gospel songs. The best part of the walk for me was that my daughter and I got to do the walk together. It was also wonderful to see around 10,000 people supporting the cause of breast cancer.

I was asked by a "friend" if I thought, "God gave me breast cancer so I would learn to love my breasts?" I do not even remember my answer to her question. I probably was too shocked by her rude question to even answer. But I do know breast cancer has helped me appreciate my breasts and many other things in life which I took for granted. The lessons learned and the people who have been so dear to me have made my journey less painful and my life fuller and brighter. Yes I may get an occasional dumb question thrown my way. But if I dodge the dumb questions and dwell on the good things people have done and said I think I will be a much happier person. I think this quote from www.livehappy.com says it all, "Protect your spirit from contamination. Limit your time with negative people." In the long run the good outweighs the bad. What more can we ask for out of life?

An Update on What I Am
Doing Now

*A*FTER MUCH CONSIDERATION I decided to have tattoos put on my breast cancer scars because I wanted to smile when I looked in the mirror instead of frown. I really could not talk myself into going through anymore surgeries. I found a tattoo artist by the name of Constance Payne. She does amazing tattoos and is a digital media specialist. The first time I met her I was impressed with her sense of humor, her amazing studio and clever jewelry made out of bugs. We sent messages back and forth on Facebook her asking me what ideas I had and me responding with pictures. I also texted Constance a picture of a flower design from a purse my sister had recently sent me and I told her I wanted to put this flower design where my nipples should be. She loved the idea and so in our first two hour session I left her studio with flowers for nipples. We recently did another session which lasted four hours and she tattooed flowers on my scars. She designed all my tattoos on her own, with a few suggestions here and there from me. During the tattoo sessions Constance makes me laugh. She tells me about her life and I tell her about mine. Before I started the tattoos I warned Constance I may cry the entire time because I felt it may be very emotional for me to change my scars to beautiful works of art. Who knows I may cry from happiness because every session brings me closer to beautiful breasts. Constance has made me feel comfortable topless and scarred. When I look in the mirror I cannot stop smiling. How could I not smile when I see flower nipples? I will always love her for making me smile. It has not only made me smile my friends seem to like the results too. When I went to lunch with my friends Roberta and Jean they insisted I show them my tattoos. They loved them and raved about how well Constance covered up my scars. So thank you again Constance. I love you and your creativity. I found a quote that says it all, "I do not need therapy I just need to talk to my tattoo artist," Funny Quotes via Facebook.

I currently am separated after 38 years of marriage. I live in my little beach house in Florida. When I think of this enormous changes which have occurred in my life I think of this quote, "Everyone has gone through something which has changed them in a way that they could never go back to the person they once were." Unknown

I found a local GYN who is wonderful. His name is Dr. Cortez and he also has a wonderful sense of humor. When I warned him about my recently acquired nipple tattoos, he stopped a minute before he opened my gown to do a breast exam. Then he proceeded to open the gown and chuckle, "You do have tattoos don't you?" I am so lucky I found a doctor who has a sense of humor which is very important to me because I love to laugh and I need a doctor that loves to laugh also. After we finished the exam he said I needed to see an oncologist and he recommended one for me to see. Since I was seeing an oncologist every year in Ohio he said I needed to find one in Florida. A couple of weeks later I meet with the oncologist and to my surprise he said, "You had pre-cancer not cancer so I do not need to see you again. Your GYN will be able to take care of any issues you have." So once again I was being pushed aside and treated like I did not belong in the "breast cancer circle." When I go back to see my Florida GYN it will be interesting to get his take on why the oncologist does not feel he needs to see me again. I wonder when things will change for women like me. I hope anyone who has had my type of breast disease or as I call it "cancer" will contact me and tell me their story. It will be interesting to see how our situations are similar and if we experienced the same "doctor problems."

Helping others makes me forget my problems and it makes me feel like a better person. I currently volunteer for the local Vitas Hospice program. I do TAP phone calls and bereavement calls to check on Hospice patients and their families. I also do home visits. At these visits I sit with a patient for about an hour once a week. It gives their caretakers a chance to have a break and it gives the patient a new face to see every week. I also hope to get a dog soon so that I can be a part of their pet program. This program brings animals to visit Hospice patients. Volunteering makes me feel good about myself and I choose to volunteer at Hospice because I had cancer and because they were so much help to my brother Timmy who died because of his cancer.

Another benefit of living in Florida is I get to see my sister Gail. I live only three hours away from her. I hope we will be close since we did not get a chance to know each other when we were growing up. She invited me to spend my birthday at her house so I drove down to see her and her husband. The first night she had the neighbors and their kids come over after dinner. The neighbor kid and I celebrated our joint birthday together with a cake and ice cream party. After we had the party Gail and I went to check out her little town and we walked, talked and drank martinis at a local bar. The next day we went to a Zac Brown Band concert and then on Sunday they took me for a ride on their boat with their two sweet dogs. We ended the visit with lunch by the river at an amazing restaurant. She and her husband were so good to me that weekend and I had so much fun. What a great way to spend birthday number 57!

Gail and I also did a road trip on Mother's Day weekend to visit my adopted mother (Gail's Aunt). We decided our road trip was going to be more than a drive from point A to point B. Instead we stopped at anything along the way which looked like fun. We stopped and took a picture of Gail standing in front of a 30 foot metal rooster. We went on a glass bottom boat ride and we stopped at St. Mark's lighthouse. We had so much fun when we got to our destination we felt like we had been on vacation. The next morning we went to church with my mom. After church we went to a High Tea at a local Tea room, where my mom had made reservations. My mom fell in love with Gail and I feel like she and I are becoming more than sisters we are becoming friends. My mother also loves having Gail in her life she asked me to give her phone number and address to Gail. Gail has a love of live and a joy for life which is very contagious. Her daughter Amanda has been sweet too, she texts me and sends me messages via Facebook. She has also invited me to spend Christmas with her, her husband and two children. It will be wonderful to share Christmas with my new family, I feel lucky because I have found a new branch of my family.

Family is very important and now that I am living in Florida I have been lucky enough to be with various members of my family. My oldest sister bought my old car from me. I drove it to my mother's house in Florida where my sister was staying. It was a nice trip even though I was alone. It made me realize I should go visit my mom more often. The next day my sister, her boyfriend and my mother and I took off for Ohio. We stopped and visited my brother's widow and spent the night at her house. We visited Timmy's grave and then stopped by my daughter Jessie's house and visited with her, her husband David and my wonderful grandson Caleb. The trip was so much fun and I felt so close to my family. When they dropped me off in Kentucky at Jessie's house and went on to Ohio I really missed them. The decision to join them on their trip was a last minute decision on my part. The trip was a blessing God gave me and now-a-days when he gives me these blessings I snatch them up and run with them. During my visit to Ohio I got to swim with my grandson Caleb. I was excited to try out the new swimsuits which camouflage my breast issues (one side is bigger than the other). I can proudly say I wore my swimsuit without feeling awkward or self-conscious. The swimsuits make me feel good on the outside and knowing I have tattoos covering my breast scars makes me feel good on the inside. During my visit I also got to give Caleb a bath, read him a bedtime story and put him to bed. I have to confess when he cried (because he does not like to go to bed) and said "Bye." I had to kiss him and run out of the room because I knew it was the last time I would put him to bed or even see him for a while. I dropped to the floor in the hall and cried my heart out. Sometimes even the joys in life tear at our hearts because we do not want to let them go. We want to hold on to them and keep the joy going on and on. The memories of that wonderful trip will forever make me smile. I also got to visit my Ohio friends: Jean, Roberta and Paula. So I thank God for the last minute trip which turned out to be the trip of a lifetime. When I flew back alone and got home with only my cats to greet me I felt a little lonely. I truly believe Florida is where God wants me to be and I will work to make it a happy place.

Living in Florida has a lot of good things going for it. I now attend church and am a member of several meet-up groups. I have also tried dating via Match.com and went on four dates. I am currently dating a man I met on the Zoosk dating site. I feel like every date teaches me more about myself and is an experience I need to go through. I found this quote on Facebook and it is going to be my mantra: "Three grand essentials to happiness in this life are something to do, something to love and something to hope for," Joseph Addison.

Volunteering for Hospice brings me happiness and I have met some wonderful people who also volunteer. I love living in Florida but I miss seeing my grandson Caleb and my daughter Jessie. I keep them in my heart. I love my grandson so much some days I struggle with the longing to see him and I cannot stop crying. I joined a writing group so I could write and get these heavy feelings out of my heart and onto paper. At one of the meetings I wrote this story about the deep longing I have to see my grandson Caleb:

The Merry-Go-Round

As Caleb and I whirled around on the Merry-Go-Round his eyes got big and he held on tight as the speed accelerated. I had not seen him in two months so it made me happy to watch the expression on his little face and listen to him engage in his toddler babble.

I tried to quiet the nagging voice in my head that kept saying, "You only get to see him for a couple of hours then you will not see him again for months." I wanted to shush the voice and embrace the few hours I had to spend with him. Because he was my only grandchild it made me feel very vulnerable.

I wanted to see him every week not every few months. But I now live over 800 miles away. The thought of the long distance miles between us left me fuming. I needed to stop worrying about the future and embrace these moments with my one year-old grandson.

Life was great so I decided to enjoy this moment in time. I grabbed his hand and we ran off to the next adventure we would find at the mall.

I loved writing that story about Caleb and how much I miss him. I also miss my friends in Ohio and I miss everything I had in my life for 56 years in Ohio. Life does not always turn out like you think it will. It does not mean life is not going just like God wants it to go. His plans for me were not the plans I had laid out for my life. In my heart I know his plans will be better.

I want to end with this wonderful quote from Mother Teresa: "People are often unreasonable and self-centered. Forgive them anyway. If you are kind, people may accuse you of ulterior motives. Be kind anyway. If you are honest, people may cheat you. Be honest anyway. If you find happiness, people may be jealous. Be happy anyway. The good you do today may be forgotten tomorrow. Do good anyway. Give the world the best you have and it may never be enough. Give your best anyway. For you see, in the end, it is between you and God. It was never between you and them anyway."

Acknowledgements

I WANT TO thank Angelina Jolie for letting people know a double mastectomy does not make one less of a woman! Thanks to my adopted mother, Mary for taking me in when she already had four children to raise.

Thanks to both of my daughters for giving me such joy by just being you. I love you both more than you will ever know.

I want to thank my daughter Shawndra for being brave enough to give up everything and take a chance on becoming a writer.

I want to thank my daughter Jessica for giving me a precious grandson to love and cherish. Nana is so much in love with Caleb! I see so much of little Jessie in him which makes me love him even more.

Thanks to both my son-in-laws for helping me move to Florida and for loving my daughters and being good husbands and friends to them.

Thanks to my marriage/divorce counselor, Elizabeth, some weeks I only survived because of you!

Thanks to all my friends and relatives for helping me in the many ways you have with your support laughter and love.

Thanks to my niece Angie for being my divorce lawyer (not legally but close enough) and a listening ear.

Thanks to my sister Gail we are making a whole lifetime of memories together.

Thanks to Mike you have brought happiness to my life that I was not expecting.

Thanks to my first Florida friend Sandie for giving a shoulder to cry on when I need it.

Thanks to God for giving me the ocean to walk beside every day. I not only feel his presence when I walk by the beach I also see the glorious beauty he has created for me and the whole world to enjoy! "My Presence watches over you continually. I have engraved you on the palm of My hands," Jesus Calling. Thanks to God for holding me in the palm of his hand and keeping me safe.

www.ingramcontent.com/pod-product-compliance
Lightning Source LLC
Chambersburg PA
CBHW020526290526
45786CB00002B/767